How I Healed
My Mind

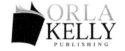

ORLA
KELLY
PUBLISHING

By Lucy Devine

Contents

Overview

How I Healed My Mind is book two in a trilogy of books I have interpreted and written since 2004. My Invisible World is the first book in this trilogy. I am currently writing my third book, Healing through Light Awareness.

In a dream in 2004, a spirit handed me a book called The Annals of Healing. I have only recently realised that it downloaded into my sensory awareness. It has revealed itself as the inspiration and bright Light that lit up the pathways during my healing journey as I travel into the hidden darkness of my mind, emotions, religion, and pain. The books revealed all the invisible and unknown in my mind that manifested as the controlling and driving forces that urged me to survive, but also created my unknown, invisible paralysing pain.

During the exploration of my mind, I interpreted that the mind is not the brain, though it is greatly supported and influenced by the brain. It is an energy-based complexity of cells that can be altered, released and healed through Light awareness without using drugs of any description.

Above all, I have discovered my higher self, which is the Light within my heart. I have recreated my mind into this enlightened reality of Light awareness that permits me to self-heal and meditate from this resource.

I hope when you read my books, you may find points that resonate in your mind, which may help identify why you need to begin to self-heal and build awareness by connecting with your higher self, your Light within.

The consequences of receiving inadequate healings remain not with the inadequate healer, but with the person who receives such healing.

After their healing, the person soon realises that they are feeling the powerlessness of darkness, as all sorts of overwhelming emotions are revealed in their minds, particularly feelings of hurt or previously unknown fears. Their healer has not informed them how or what to do with these feelings.

When you begin your healing journey, you must become aware of your Light, the higher self reality and accept the sensations of its unconditional love, which you may feel within yourself as peace, joy, freedom. From the awareness of these positive empowering feelings, the healing journey begins for most people.

Everybody needs healing. Please choose your healer carefully.

Lucy Devine

Dedicated to my sisters and brothers.

We must heal the past if we want to experience the freedom of the future.

Who am I?

I am not a wife
I am not a husband
Who am I?
I am not a sister
I have no siblings
Who am I?
I am not a daughter
I am not a son
Who am I?
I have no mother
I have no father
Who am I?
I am alive,
I am living
How do I identify
Who am I?
How do I relate,
What do I call myself?
Who am I?
"Am I not familiar to thee?"
I hear the whisper in the stillness,
My heart tremors in fear,
I deny that I know you.
Who am I?
I am Light.

Introduction

In my first book, *My Invisible World*, I began my healing journey by discovering all that was invisible and unknown to me within my mind. It opens with the question of who I am. I struggled to find answers to this question because I identified Lucy Devine from my physical reflection.

When I sought the invisible me, my higher self, the Light within my heart chakra as my reflection, I began to hear answers to my other questions about my mind, spirit, soul, emotions, and feelings. I asked who God is and why God is so difficult to find. I asked what love is, and I understood that love has many different interpretations, understandings and applications within the mind. Through my writing, I realised my love experiences were of a conditional love that created a binding force of the unsaid, the silence of the assumed within my mind and the automatically entitled thinking that fuelled pain. Above all, I discovered the invisible Light within my heart chakra was me, my higher self and my sacred connection to a higher God.

Meditation is the tool I used to open and build my awareness of the Light to my higher self reality. When I first began to meditate, I started in guided spiritual meditations that revealed the surprising, invisible realities in the most vivid colours, the most acute feelings of peace and joy, and nature's images in their purest form. I discovered my spirit guides. During this time, I explored the spirit and why spirit existed.

I was inspired during my meditations to develop an awareness of Light and recognise how it communicated with me.

My determination to seek and connect to Light eventually helped me to expand my awareness of Light. I accepted how my interpretations gradually revealed a meditation technique that helped me find the unique Light within my heart chakra.

Through this Light, I revealed my own sensory body of the aura, the chakras and the senses, and how the senses work. I discovered that the senses have a unique language that I needed to interpret.

I became aware that Light was endeavouring to heal my darkness and ignorance. My meditations inspired me to understand that I needed to work on my sensory body by aligning my chakras into a Light existence. It was the vibrancy of the Light sensations that would heal my body and my mind.

My ability to interpret Light through my senses became a gift from God for me. It was this ability to interpret Light that permitted me to grow my Light awareness existence. My Light awareness enabled me to change my perspective entirely from my learned bravado mind.

I sensed that Light is not the final destination required by me during meditation, "You need to travel further in your awareness to find God."

In this book, *How I Healed my Mind*, I discovered God, who He is, how and why I buried Him in every thought within my mind.

The Candle Flame

The candle flame I use in my life is a reflection of the highest Light vibration. The candle flame provides me with the presence of an unconditional friend as I work every day.

When I focus on the candle flame, several things occur. The candle flame provides me with a colour and structure of Light that I use in all meditations, healings, readings, and other work. The candle flame helps me unite my senses into the candle flame's single image of Light that allows me to attune to Light.

The candle flame I use in meditation provides a reflected flame of Light in the inner third eye space that enables the senses to focus upwards through this inner Light to connect to Light's highest vibration.

Focusing on the candle flame also provides the flame of Light to help the detachment process to begin. It helps me to detach from all my learning, to retrain my senses into a Light vibration, to feel my senses' Light without feeling the mind's burden, and it helps me to step a⌄ from the driving force of my thoughts that may ' ling my pain and my anxiety.

The Mechanics of My Mind

When I initially sought the mind, I closed my eyes to turn my senses inwards, hoping to see it. I could only see darkness. I relied heavily on my trust in Light and my research on the chakras for support and inspiration. The chakra system's reveal had previously inspired me to accept that my mind was a clock-like energy tool driven by the powerful chakras. I asked Light if I could see an image of the mind. I thought to myself that if I could see an image, I could work to that image. I could interpret it and begin to break it down, articulate it and express my understanding of it.

I eventually saw an image of my mind in meditation. My interpretation was that it looked similar to the moon in shape. Its energies felt soft, sponge-like in substance. I instantly remembered I had experienced a similar type of content in meditation years previously. In that meditation, I poked my head upwards to break through a thick elastic-band-type consistency of energy until it gave way, and my head went through. I could now see the mind from an ʏ̱ ̱perspective.

ᵥrance as similar to a grapefruit
ʰen it floated into my aware-
I sensed and accepted that it

was a closed vessel of energy. I needed to ask Light for help and support to open it. During another meditation, I felt inspired to open it like I would open an oyster shell. I lifted the lowest point of the shape upwards so I could see and understand its workings. I saw the inner workings to be similar to the innards of a grapefruit.

I quickly distinguished between the two parts of the skin of the grapefruit. The outer layer of skin is a film of thick, porous coloured layers with a sturdy consistency that protects the fruit from the environment. The inner part of the skin is supple white pith that encapsulates, supports and nourishes the individual cells of fruit to grow, to flourish into single fruit segments within the skin.

The mind works similarly to the grapefruit. The more robust, sturdy outer layers of the mind contain the learned powerful memories and thoughts controlled and driven by the bravado learned mind perspective.

This mind perspective automatically rejects or suppresses the subtle feelings of intuition, truth, pain and difference within itself that builds up as different layers of mainly hidden, vulnerable painful thoughts, feelings and emotions.

The bravado learned mind encapsulates the energy forces of the physical body. To help me understand this sentence, Light asked me to imagine my physical body as my hand and its skin as my mind. I found this image made it easier to see why we are not conscious of the energies of the mind. After all, I am not aware of my skin's existence unless something goes wrong and it develops a skin disease. I do not distinguish it as being separate from my body in any way. The mind is akin to an invisible skin or layer of energy that is within and around the body.

Eventually, I fully accepted my intuition about the mind when I realised that I could change and alter the dynamics of my mind. I was able to remove the power from thoughts, change them and replace them with Light-filled thoughts of awareness. I was able to unravel thought patterns that controlled my mind perspective automatically. I was able to detach from invisible dark influences that were shadowing my mind automatically. I was able to recognise, accept, engage and remove the power from emotions that enabled me to transmute them. I could break down emotions into individually created emotions and differentiate them from the inherited emotions that enabled me to recognise my unique feelings.

I detached from and healed spirits back to their original Light existences that influenced me unknowingly in negative impressions. I was also able to change and lift the mind perspective that permitted me to engage with the world from a completely different perspective.

I realised I had done all of this work on my mind through my Light perspective. I was supported in this work by Light – both in my heart chakra and universally. I realised this work did not involve or require the physical reality of my brain. I didn't need to operate on my brain to make considerable changes within my mind.

I saw that the mind's energies are power-based or powerlessly induced. When I focused on the sense of the power I had in my mind, I recognised it was thoughts of an entitled automatic desire for power.

I saw my mind strived automatically and continuously for power, money and success. I saw the powerful interactions between people as they automatically competed for power. The people I observed seemed to be winning or defeating each other in sports, conversations, debates, job interviews, politics and war. They competed in their relationships, examinations, religious opinions, and politics and in all areas of society where patriarchal law exists.

I saw that people competed even in simple conversations with each other about their absorbed and learned knowledge. They gained this knowledge from books they studied, and it automatically gave them titles of hierarchal power and influences that ruled general society. Their hierarchal power deemed their knowledge to be the primary structure that determines the dominant path to success or failure for students. This knowledge path clearly defines the right or the wrong in students' lives and the lives of people in society. The knowledge path stretches out ahead of each person as the only way that guarantees success in life. That structure places people in their deserved hierarchal place within society.

I recognised how my mind perspective automatically read people as strong and influential, and therefore, powerful. Alternatively, my perspective recognised their weaknesses, and I read this as their powerlessness or failures. I saw my ability to accept the hierarchal rules of patriarchal law and my unquestioning acceptance of a religious God's existence as a negative existence within my mind. I saw the passionate way I carried the overwhelming burdened pain of Jesus and other people as my pain during my life was dynamite in its influence on my child and adult mindsets.

I now recognise that my automatic acceptance of the existence of God and Jesus reflected in my mind society's patriarchal rule. As a child, I had no choice except to accept society's teaching and how I learned it in my school and home.

I saw that I had learned to love in the same burdensome way as I had learned to accept and love the painful images of a dying crucified Jesus. I learned to love outside of myself by reaching outwards automatically in my mind to love. I loved my mother in the silent conditioned way of society. I automatically and unquestionably believed I loved my mother in my learned and conditioned way to live and love. I recognised that this conditioned love is an assumed love and an entitled love.

Does this insight about the mind's power mean that power builds on perception and a perceived automatic acceptance of power? Does this insight mean that power is an illusion, that it is not real, and not reality?

When I initially began questioning the power of the mind, I began to question the essence of this power. In my meditations, I asked for support to differentiate between the different types of power. I asked for, and I received the colour yellow to symbolise conditioned love, conditioned thoughts, conditioned support, conditioned voices, and conditioned friendships. I also requested and received green to signify unconditional love, unconditional support, and unconditional friendship. I received the colour red as a sign of anger. These colours were clear boundaries for my initial understanding of the different powers I was separating in my mind and my relationships. My confidence and self-esteem grew. I began to trust my senses and my intuition, and I no longer needed the colours.

I began to sense the conditioned tone of the voice, the conditioned use of words, the hidden manipulation, the conditioned body language, and facial expressions that revealed the genuine truth of people's feelings. I began to detach from all of these people's power through my Light boundaries.

How did I live so long in this world and not have any understanding of the meaning of power? I accepted that my mind depended so much on power. However, was that power a reflected power? How did I not know the difference between power, reflected power, powerlessness, and empowerment?

I recognised the arrogance and ignorance of my bravado perspective did not differentiate power. Power is power, money is money, and success is demanded, entitled and expected automatically by my bravado perspective.

I began to study the reflected power of the mind. I needed to understand if the mind created power, and if so, how it happened. I needed to understand the 'want' that was a constant influence and demand in my mind.

The first perspective I unravelled was the reflected power of the mind, but I discovered various mind perspectives that I needed to recognise and unravel.

The Mind Perspectives That Piloted My Bravado Mind

The first thing I accepted about my mind was that my bravado perspective is both ignorant and arrogant of the existence of an unconditional God, Light, the aura, chakras and the universe. Therefore, the bravado mind cannot acknowledge any alternative realities except what the bravado mind knows. Whenever it hears the intuited feelings or inspired thoughts, it considers them weak and not reliable. It discards them in favour of the academic knowledge of the mind. The disregard of Light influences, which are whole in existence and empowering in vibration, created a massive void in my feelings that fuelled a vacuum of pain within my core feelings. The vacuum of pain developed the various powerless victim emotions that were either ruling me unknowingly or influencing me invisibly.

During my initial observations of the mind, I thought it grew and expanded to fit the baby's growing physical body as it advanced to adulthood. I changed my awareness when I began to understand the mechanics of the mind. The powerful bravado perspective of the mind permits the mind to expand with the growth of the body.

It has a similar capacity to restrict the mind's growth by automatically retracting its perspective to a negative, learned, invisible pain-filled mind reality.

The external challenges to a baby's newly awakened mind automatically trigger the retract mechanism that automatically spins the mind's energies into one force of energy. That force of energy is either a powerful positive or a powerless negative perspective. Either of these perspectives spin automatically into the bravado perspective. The bravado perspective fuelled by instinctual urges to survive grows the mind into a sensed power or a sensed powerlessness that automatically seeks similar vibrations of power or powerlessness, comfort or pain, familiarity or arrogance, security or defensiveness, protection or ignorance.

I saw very clearly that these images of the bravado mind arose from within the suppressed aura and the chakras, particularly at my solar plexus chakra point.

I began to trust and accept my inspiration that the mind identity is separate and apart from the brain. I started to get a sense of the original purpose of the mind. I sensed that it is an energy tool initially created by the mother's mind to protect her embryo in the womb and that it also created protection for the aura's cells.

I believe the mind is initially influenced by what it senses when the endocrine system's powerful hormones release during the different stages of growth, such as in the embryo, foetus, baby, birth journey, the newborn baby, the toddler, young child, young adult and adult. I believe that the mind interprets the sensed powerful hormones released by the endocrine system and assumes the power it senses to be the power of the mind itself. This assumption automatically generates the want for power. The want becomes the driving force of the survival mind perspective as it feels it must have the power to survive.

I began to dig deeper into the workings of the newly awakened mind for answers. I found layers of energy spinning in rotations. I started to recognise the spins as the different energy layers and their perspectives that existed in a differential existence within the powerful chakras that the bravado mind's perspective was piloting. The powerful chakras' perspectives controlled or overshadowed the weaker chakra perspectives into passive silences of compliance. The bravado perspective rotations contain the aura, chakras, and chakra systems within its circumference of control. I needed these rotations of the mind to stop for me. I needed to unravel the circumference of energies before I could begin the healing of my mind. I started my healing by stopping these rotations.

I intuited how to begin my healing in meditation by realigning my chakras, by applying my grounding and detachment boundaries to the mind's circumference. This realignment of the chakras became a primary function of the healing process for me.

My research revealed the three invisible existences within the mind that are paramount in understanding how the mind creates. They are the invisible chakras, the hidden unique interpreted truth sensed by the foetus's aura in the womb, and my unique ability to interpret sensory truth and suppress it automatically in favour of a learned conditioned truth.

The First Invisible Existence

I will begin with a description of the first invisible existence, the spinning reality of the invisible chakras. I will describe how the chakras form the basic structure of the mind.

The Solar Plexus

The first most powerful perspective within the Bravado Mind

(It contains or eclipses the existence of the heart chakra)

The solar plexus chakra is the all-powerful chakra of learned knowledge that believes its existence is the only existence, the highest existence, the powerful existence to how humanity should live.

The solar plexus chakra is the generator of power that combines the mind and body's energies as a single force of power. This powerful mindset thrives on a single intentioned purpose of academia, including learning how to accept conditioned and learned love as the only love. Its powerful knowledge automatically promotes its existence to be the most powerful and only reality for humanity. I saw that the glory of power made this mindset the highest point of achievement, and in essence, it becomes the 'brain' of the mind. This powerfulness protects the mind. It also ensures it remains closed to all other external influences except those acceptable and compatible with the all-powerful learned knowledge mindset.

The solar plexus perspective automatically captures and suppresses the existence of the Light within the heart chakra.

The Light of the Heart Chakra
The First Overshadowed Chakra of the Bravado Mind

The Light of the heart chakra is the centre of all our feelings and sensations of unconditional love. The existence of this unique flame of Light provides an automatic connection to the higher Light of the universe for the human being. I accept the heart chakra is known to be the seat of Light consciousness, which is the higher self within each human being. The heart chakra's existence is captured or eclipsed by the solar plexus power whose perspective conditions humans to believe and accept conditional love as the one love, the pure and only love of both God and man.

However, the Light of the heart chakra is the embodiment of unconditional love. The seeker can access it by seeking it through the senses. I found it necessary to use my Light boundaries to detach from the powerful solar plexus chakra perspective.

The perspective of the Light of the heart chakra is of unconditional love, compassion and empathy.

The Sacral Chakra

The Second Chakra of the Bravado Mind

(This overshadows the Throat Chakra)

The sacral chakra is the second perspective of the Bravado Mind that automatically conforms to the solar plexus mind forces.

It is the centre of natural physical creativeness in that both the male and the female carry their reproductive organs within the energies of this chakra. For this reason, I make this chakra the powerful centre for physical creation and the continuance of the human race.

This chakra perspective is usually a passive or an unknown angry perspective because it inspires a powerful mental denial mechanism nurtured by the solar plexus perspective of powerlessness that contains the suppressed, denied, or inherited unfamiliar emotions. The denial mechanism of this chakra is not the human's ability to reproduce babies. That assumption is an unquestioned automatic entitlement in the bravado mindset of both sexes. The denial mechanism lies in the fundamental lack of acceptance of the core values of the higher self. The denial of the unique self makes the inherited emotions and the learned self the person's identity.

The void of an internal lacking nurtured the bravado barriers in my mindset of irresponsibility, recklessness, and assumed arrogance to life generally. I was also ignorant of any sense of responsibility in my femininity and my sexuality. I was very much an identity of my learning, of my crippling intuition, unexpressed emotions and the acceptance of my inherited emotions.

The sacral chakra perspective in all of its entitled assumptions and knowledge automatically suppresses, dismisses, or denies the throat chakra's existence.

Throat Chakra

The Second Overshadowed Chakra of the Bravado Mind

The throat chakra is the second overshadowed chakra. It is the centre of our unique expression of truth that is the voice of the aura. It is the voice of Light, the expression of unconditional love.

The throat chakra perspective is that of truth, compassion and empathy.

The weighted knowledge of the solar plexus and the sacral chakra perspectives automatically suppress this chakra's unique truth. Instead, the human being learns to speak the learned truth. The learned truth is what must be said to please influential people. The learned truth becomes the truth, becomes the identity until we, as individuals, decide to seek and find the unique truth by detaching and healing the learned barriers that choke this chakra. It is necessary to use the Light boundaries to detach from the learning of the solar plexus and sacral chakra mindsets to engage the voice of this chakra, the voice and expression of the truth of Light.

The Base Chakra

The Third Chakra perspective of the Bravado Mind

(It overshadows the third eye chakra)

The base chakra is the third chakra perspective of the Bravado Mind that automatically conforms to the solar plexus perspective.

This powerful learned mindset generates from the internal learning and silent interpretations that build automatically to create the learned reflected identity of the human mind. The perspective of the base chakra mindset is that of a learned survival mind perspective. The internal learning and the silent interpretations of this chakra are burdened and influenced by the weighted knowledge of the solar plexus and the sacral chakras mindsets.

It was from this chakra perspective I learned to internalise my feelings and thoughts as a small child. I learned to survive mentally, emotionally and spiritually from this chakra perspective. From this place of immature learning in my mind, I grew into the reflected mindset that flourished in the approval or disapproval of the family dynamic and society. I interpreted and intuitively learned to love from adults. I interpreted how to gain their approval and how to deal with their disapproval. I learned to please them, to be obedient to them and society. I learned to accept adult behaviour as right. I learned dutiful thoughts. I learned dependency on other people. I automatically developed an unknown bravado anger barrier to protect myself from adults. All this interpreting and learning were the fundamental basics of my mind for most of my life until I changed my thinking when I began my self-healing.

The identity of the base chakra determines the automatic expression of knowledge and learning. It reflects the automatic behaviour consciously, subconsciously, unconsciously, and sexually.

Generally, this childlike bravado perspective reflects the power of the penis and its dominant influences in our society, as does the power of the vagina and the womb. The penis, which determines the future of the human race on Planet Earth, can also be a weapon of entitlement in either mindset.

The power of this chakra's entitlement is reflected in the human mind when a person demands to fulfil their sexual wants without consideration for rights or free will and whose entitled behaviour is supported by a patriarchal entitled society. The automatic want for sexual gratifications reflects a conditioned learned knowledge of love with little or no self-esteem for either of the sexes. When I realigned the base chakra, I found it a chakra that supported my interpretative skills as I built my unique sensory awareness.

Third Eye Chakra

The Third Overshadowed Chakra of the Bravado Mind

In its original true essence of Light, the third eye chakra is the all-seeing, all-powerful sensory connection to Light. It has automatic anchorage to the Light of the universe that supports and influences it. It is also this Light that is the consistent link between all humans.

The third eye mind perspective is perception. When the third eye perspective works through the power of the three previous chakras, its perception will be of spiritually and religiously influenced learned knowledge. When the third eye works through a Light perspective, it becomes the all-knowing and the all-seeing perspective that is all influential and empowering.

A person's life journey begins with the generation of the Light of their aura that is automatically rebooted to a mental consciousness of darkness as the baby is born. I believe this forty-week journey in the womb and the birth journey becomes the journey of a lifetime for a person's mind.

It provides each human with an identity of either male or female and with the fundamental automatic ability to survive. The survival existence is the lowest point of living because it invisibly influences minds, mainly in fear that self-generates invisible pain. This hidden pain eventually becomes the high price of suffering to both the mind and the body as they break down into sickness, illness, and disease.

When a person seeks Light influences through this chakra, instant healing is achievable. This healing will also help release the remembered and fearful shadows of spirit automatically retained in thoughts and memories that influence the bravado perspective.

The Feet Chakras

The Fourth and Fifth Chakras perspectives of the Bravado Mind

(They overshadow the Crown chakra)

The feet chakras are the fourth and fifth perspectives of the Bravado Mind that automatically conform to the solar plexus and align to society's collective perspectives.

The bravado mind perspective of the feet chakras finds its resources of power in their external connections to the energies of the collective consciousness. These chakras carry the power of personal intention, whether that is an individual conscious intention or the intention of the collective consciousness.

The feet chakras perspective enables the spinning of the bravado mind automatically.

I did not know about the feet chakras until I began my self-healing. They were revealed to me by Light to help in my evolving process. I saw that through the existence of these chakras, I started the detachment process from my bravado mind. I also began grounding my Light awareness into the earth, which helped me to feel secure and authentic in my sensory self. The detachment boundary tool allowed me to separate my Light awareness from the powerful bravado collective mind dynamic. I began to reveal the powerless internal aspects of my hurt self.

When I realigned the feet chakras into their proper positions, they were pivotal in revealing the exit points necessary for Light to enter the ground to complete the grounding boundary. The detachment process permitted me to realign all the chakras to the Light awareness of my heart chakra and attune my senses to my Light wisdom.

The Crown Chakra

The Fourth overshadowed Chakra of the Bravado Mind

The crown chakra is the fourth overshadowed perspective of the Bravado Mind that automatically conforms to the solar plexus forces.

The crown chakra's perspective is that of a religious or spiritual opinion that reflects the learning of the bravado mind.

In a correctly aligned chakra system, the crown chakra is at the top of the head, and its channel enables the Light in the heart chakra and the entire chakra system to connect and remain connected to the Light of the universe.

Unfortunately, the feet chakras collective perspective has made this chakra the connection point to a religious or spiritual God. From this perspective, people connect to the collective existences of the invisible, unknown spirit world at the lowest point in the mind, at the feet vibrations.

When I discovered my feet chakras perspectives, I discovered my senses connected to the image of a religious, conditional, righteous, suffering God. My connection to this God was from a place of learned humility, suffering and loss. From this place in my mind, I discovered I also connected to the spirit existence to facilitate my healing career. How can I make a positive connection to anyone from the pained place of a bowed head, on my knees, with closed eyes in the full knowledge of suffering? How was I going to heal myself or anyone else from this mind perspective? Within myself, I saw this image of total passivity and a learned conditioned humility fuelled my mind perspective in a downward spiral into various spiritual vibrations of pain in the great collective consciousness of society. This chakra became the seal of spiritual energies that set the bravado perspective to a collective consciousness dynamic.

The chakras dynamic was the first invisible and unknown part of my mind that Light revealed to me. The reveal of the fundamentals of my invisible, unknown dark mind was where my mind's healing began for me.

The Second Invisible Existence

The second invisible and unknown reality that Light revealed to me was the existence of the hidden unique interpreted truth sensed by the foetus's aura during the gestation period in the womb.

The truth of these sensations is pivotal in determining the vibrations the mind activates at, as it awakens when the baby separates physically from its mother. Nevertheless, the hidden truth becomes the invisible magnet of a sensed influential pain that is the hidden truth of unknown memories and contained hidden painful emotions. This magnet was a force of pain within my mind that influenced me in the darkness of invisible pain that was a significant negative power physically, mentally, emotionally, and spiritually.

The Third Invisible Existence

The third invisible and unknown reality that Light revealed to me was my unique ability to interpret sensory truth and suppress it automatically in favour of a learned conditioned truth.

Sensory truth is the truth of Light, and my interpreted sensory truth is unique to me. I can interpret what I sense into thoughts and feelings in my mind. The bravado mind automatically denies or contains the sensory truth favouring the power of the learned conditioned truth. The learned conditioned truth begins its growth when the baby is born and begins a physical relationship with its mother.

The baby learns how to feel that will flourish into emotions and memories that become the everyday reality within the baby's mind. These learned feelings will mirror the mother's mindset and the mindset of the family dynamic.

These learned feelings may reveal as:

- The baby may sense aloneness and cries for the comfort of love but will learn from its mother's actions and responses. As she soothes her baby with food, food becomes a comfort for the baby.
- Similarly, the baby feels lonely and cries to gain the comfort of love from its mother. The baby learns to memorise loneliness as hunger because the mother feeds her baby to stop the crying.
- When the baby feels fear and cries to gain the comfort of love from its mother, she feeds it food to stop the crying. Hence the baby may learn fear is hunger and learns comfort from food.
- A baby senses the darkness and cries for the attention and love of its mother. The mother believes in not spoiling her baby and leaves it to cry out. As a result, her baby will develop fear and identifies fear as love.
- A newborn baby feels rejected by the mother and cries for reassurance and love. The mother believes in not spoiling the baby and leaves it to cry out. As a result, the baby learns the feelings that align with isolation and rejection.
- The baby and mother are separated, the baby cries to reconnect with her, but she does not respond to her baby's cries. The baby learns and memorises feelings that align with rejection, isolation and abandonment.

This internal sensing and learning of a baby build the mindset of its learning. The mind grows into the learning of conditioned love in the child-mind. The conditioned love builds into a mask that hides the unknown internal interpretation of truth and the fear of truth in all its guises.

Conditional love is the invisible, unknown, silent, unsaid, binding love between mother and child. It fuels the growing mind's automatic survival perspective to be silent, unquestioning, obedient and dutiful. It feeds the child-mind to be robotic in its acceptance of actions and reactions as a love that may involve parents' brutal physical and mental actions. Conditioned love becomes the invisible yet powerful perspective in a child/adult's mind. It will become apparent to the mind of the growing child/ young adult, to parents and peers as the child begins to build relationships. The child/young adult's relationships with the family dynamic and other people will reveal the extent of pain in their automatic mind perspective.

I found these unknown existences during my healing revelations. It was in my acceptance of these revelations that I found and understood my chronic pain. This reveal was pivotal in finding my sensory Light, my higher self and living my life firmly grounded in my Light perspective.

I feel this completes the unknown, invisible existences within the mind that reflect the void, the chasm that determines the vibration of a person's mind. Upon this invisibility of the 'unknown' and 'invisible,' the bravado mind grows and flourishes, mainly in power and pain. I was accepting that the quest for power mainly creates pain. This pain automatically builds as a powerless void within. The powerless void perspective within always seeks its perception of power.

After this study of revelations, I began to ask where the real power of the mind exists.

I remember looking at men and wondering if their minds worked in the same way as my mind. Did they sense powerlessness in the same way I did? I was trying to sort out for myself if men and women were equal to each other. I asked God if men and women were equal, why did he not create us in the same body without the differences between male and female? I wondered if we are not equal in the physical body, are we equal in our minds?

I interpreted the answers to these questions by understanding that I needed to break down the difference between power, perceived power, and reflected power. I also needed to understand the difference between the mind and the brain.

I began by separating the energies of the mind from the brain. Then I separated the brain energies from the third eye chakra. I then separated the third eye energies from spirit existences and influences.

Now, I had four separate components to the mind that operated through the single bravado mind perspective:

1. The Third Eye Chakra: the individual connection to the Light of the universe.
2. The Mind: the energy mass that is the individually created, unique mind dynamic.

3. Spirit.
4. The Brain: the individual physical organ of the body.

1. The Third Eye Chakra

In my meditation, I heard God designed the brain precisely to encapsulate the third eye Light forces. Through its encapsulation of Light, the brain transforms itself into a powerful generator that produces power from Light energies. The generator is unaware of the existence of the third eye chakra. It purposely drives the Light of the third eye chakra, along with all the other chakras, to fuel the different functions silently, effortlessly, and efficiently that keeps the body functioning and healthy.

2. The Mind

I began to articulate from my interpretations that the mind's creation begins with the aura that generates a very high Light energy at conception. For the duration of the pregnancy and indeed, through life, it continually vibrates as it absorbs, transmits and retains interpreted information through its heightened senses. The interpreted sensations remain in the aura's cells and only develop into layers of the inner mind during the baby's birth. The inner mind crystallises into an invisible, unknown vibration that happens when its sensed information becomes thoughts and feelings. The whole mind awakens as the baby is born and separates from the mother.

The outer bravado survival mind creates lower vibrations than the aura. It manifested for me as the tough exterior four layers of energies generated by the mother's bravado mind during her pregnancy.

I observed the **first layer of energies** wrapped around the aura of the embryo in the womb. They are the organic retentive energies powered by the mother's endocrine system to retain the embryo within her womb. The womb's energies automatically create a secure and comforting, supportive layer of energy for the embryo to sense and feel until the baby is born. These retentive layers of energies powered by the mother's endocrine system to retain the embryo within her womb make up the first layer of encompassing energy.

The **second layer of energies** I observed surrounding the embryo in the womb, generates from the mother's intuitive automatic urgings from her heart to protect and keep her embryo safe. This second layer of energies generates from her protective feelings of love, her automatic and intuitive intention to protect her embryo. This layer of energies encompasses the previous layer of energies.

The **third layer of energies** generates from the mother's energies of her internal mental thinking that automatically projects and transmits her inner thoughts and feelings freely to her embryo's energies. It projects her subconscious and unconscious thoughts and feelings, her thoughts and feelings of her practised religious and spiritual beliefs. I observed that this energy layer encompasses the previous two layers of energies surrounding the embryo in the womb. I saw that this third layer of energies retained and absorbed the mother's bravado mind throughout the pregnancy in a passive, non-responsive way. It is the third layer of mind energies generated by the mother's bravado mind. I accepted that this layer of energies expanded into the mother aspect of the baby's mind when it awakened at birth.

I also observed the **fourth layer of energies** generated from the mother's unique interpretations of the energy transmissions of the words and feelings that flow freely between her and her baby's father. She interprets her unique truth about her man, the father of her baby, in her silent inner mind. She intuitively interprets his powerfulness, his behaviour, his thoughts and thinking, his survival skills, his coping skills, his successes, his failures, his weaknesses, his moods and his tone of voice. She automatically transmits her interpretations to generate the fourth layer of energies that encompass her foetus as it grows in the womb. This survival layer of energies will absorb the sensations of the endocrine systems of the baby/mother when they release powerful adrenaline into the body of the unborn baby to activate and motivate it to be born.

It is the fourth layer of energies generated by the mother's mindset and is her interpretation of the male survival energies. This energy layer forms the primary survival energies that will eventually expand to become the father aspect of the baby's mind when it awakens at birth. This reveal was a tremendous insight for me to both comprehend and articulate.

I needed to understand what happens to these layers of energies during the birth journey of the baby. While still in the womb, I saw the baby's endocrine system fire up in unison with the mother's endocrine system. The combined endocrine systems release the powerful hormones of adrenaline that begin the birthing journey. The baby reacts to these surges of power it feels within itself by pushing outwards from the womb through the birth canal. The mother supports the baby's efforts by pushing the baby out of her body. The baby's journey of darkness through a tiny tunnel triggers multiple sensations of feelings in its awareness. The combined forces of adrenaline power drive the baby to be born and register in the baby's mind as its experiences of power and the drive to survive. I believe this sensed driving power is the 'want' for power that grows into the bravado survival-based mind.

I accept that the bravado survival-based mind perspective does not create its power, but it relies on the memories of sensed power and its perception of power. The sensed power and the perceived power perspectives reveal in a person's thoughts, feelings and emotions. I believe the mind is survival-based energy cells and is created on the interpretations of memorised sensed power searching for the reality of a memorised feeling of power.

I list the different thinking that explains the sensed power, perceived power, reflected power, and powerlessness.

i.   The mind automatically uses the unknown, the invisible connection to the universal power, as its power. The universal power breaks down as the aspect of Light, the unique Light of the person, the muted hidden Light of the aura, and the chakra system. We recognise this power in our thinking as we automatically think the brain is the ultimate powerful mind. The brain identifies as a person that controls and protects both the mind itself and the body.

ii.   The mind automatically uses the invisible connections to the different planets within the universe as its power. We can recognise this power in our complete, entitled reliance and dependence on the cycles of the sun, moon and the stars for our survival. We have further automatic reliance on the universal planets that influence us unconditionally. In our minds, we take and accept these influences as a unique power. For example, an astrology chart will inform anyone who asks which planets were in sync and aligned when they were born. The information the astrology chart provides is a potent influence within the mind. We absorb the power of this influence automatically as our identity, strength, mind dynamic, and beauty without acknowledging its value or its source from within the universe.

iii. The mind automatically uses its reflected learning power, particularly the remembered power gained from the knowledge retained in the subconscious mind. We can recognise the power of authors who have written learned knowledge in 'successful' books chosen by our schools, libraries, colleges, and universities to influence humanity's minds in a specific collective dynamic of learning. From these institutional perspectives, we evaluate our population in accreditations. These same accreditations determine success and failure and place individuals in the different hierarchy levels within the reflected power of collective society.

iv. The mind uses the power it perceives from the powerful dynamic of our community and society's collective thinking. We can recognise this reflected power in our automatic admiration towards influential, powerful people and our imitation of their behaviour and thinking.

v. The mind automatically uses the power of the inherited and conditioned mind perspectives of past generations. It is an entitled power that descendant families claim as their right, their entitlement. Their superior positions upheld automatically in the hierarchal places of power within societies. The human being automatically defaults to their place in society's hierarchal power as we accept without question the power in titles, lineage and money, and the automatic acceptances and entitlements of the financial inheritances of this lineage.

vi.   The mind accepts the collective power of religion. Religion's conditioned judgemental opinions automatically eclipse a person's unique power into powerlessness of passive thinking or even sacrificial thinking. We automatically obey the religious rule that tells us how we should live our lives. We accept their rigid influence in our education system. We obey and follow their strict laws on how we should marry, their unrelenting opinions on how we should rear our children, and finally, on how we should die.

vii.   The mind uses the perceived power of a conditioned religious hierarchy and its deity. We carry an automatic blind dependence and reliance on faith and belief in God's reflective invisible images and their messengers. Our faith in them is firm in our minds without understanding their source or where they come from, or the need for personal boundaries of protection from spiritual pain.

3. Spirit

I speak in this section of the powerful unknown influences spirit had in my mind.

I inherited my silent automatic interpretation of the spiritual influences from my family and my community. From a young, innocent age, I learned my immature interpretations and understanding of religion that became very influential in my adult mind. I recognised the devastating unquestioning painful application these influences had in and on my mind. I found its pain in my bravado perspective, thoughts, passive and thwarted emotions. It also revealed in my body as chronic pain that pierced the frozen parts of my body – spine, hips, limbs, joints, organs.

I also speak here of the unknown, invisible spirit identities I found snuggled up in the painful vibrations of my mind during my meditations. My mind's low vibrations were in acute pain, and the spirit existences were in similar pain. My pain supported these spirit's realities automatically and unknowingly in their suffering. They felt comforted and supported emotionally and spiritually in my pain vibrations. Their spiritual and mental drive to survive aligned with my mind's purpose to survive. The reveal of these spirit existences and how they worked after their physical bodies' death was another shocking acceptance for me. Their invisible presence and influences within my mind were not of my choosing and were unknown to me.

However, their low and pained vibrations influenced me in darkened shadows. Their driving needs to survive attached to my survival-based mind. Their pain and trauma charged and fed my invisible chronic pain. These influences were unknown to me and everyone else. They emerged as my unexplained irrational emotions that influenced my chronic pain that was affecting my body.

I revealed them in my unredeemed sense of loss that I could not fill. I revealed their layers in the perceived passive emotional reality that I could not control or quench in my mind.

All of this irrational and paranoid drama kept my mind perspective suspicious, distrustful, angry, and cynical. The reveal of these spirits and their influences in my mind only occurred after I released the way I connected and related to my religious God and its hierarchy of deity.

4. The Brain

I took the brain and observed it as it encapsulated the third eye chakra Light forces. I saw instantly that the brain turned into a powerful generator that had a dual purpose.

The first purpose revealed how it automatically charged the Light energies of the third eye chakra and the entire chakra system into a powerful energy force.

The second purpose revealed how the brain pumped this energy around the body.

Below I have listed out all the recognisable functions the brain performs every second of every minute of every day that keeps the physical body functioning healthy and alive. For example, the brain generator powers and drives the following energy systems that, in turn, drive the physical body into a living state.

1. The nervous system
2. The circulation system
3. The digestive system

4. The respiratory system
5. The lymphatic system
6. The muscular system
7. The reproductive system
8. The endocrine system
9. The immune system
10. The skeletal system
11. The Skin

All of these functions of the brain are essential to the working of the mind and the body. I found the most potent brain function to be the function of the endocrine system. It plays a hugely important, mainly invisible and spectacularly powerful role within the human being, the brain itself and the human mind. The endocrine gland is the hypothalamus, classified as part of the brain. It directly controls the pituitary gland and has an indirect impact on the other glands of the endocrine system.

The pineal gland (also within the brain) is a very powerful gland that determines our sexuality, development, and expansion. The pineal gland's power determines, not just our sexuality, but also defines our growth physically and our development as human beings. I understand many diseases in the body are based here in the centre of the endocrine system.

I revealed that the brain I had previously understood to be my mind and my identity for most of my life was not my mind. When I separated the brain from the Light of the third eye and all the other invisible energies, the brain is just a dead muscle.

I can see that I lost 'me' in the constant want for power from my bravado perspective. I forgot the awareness of my Light consciousness entirely that is the most sacred component of who I am.

It has become my mission to reclaim these suppressed cells back to the Light and to align them with the intention of God, free from the void of pain, shadow, the automatic want for power, memories of survival, the inherited mind dynamic, the appetite for power, the perception of power, and the projection of power.

I feel I am only beginning to understand the impact the endocrine system has on the human being. When I found the endocrine system, I began to sense the energy differences between man and woman.

The Endocrine System

I interpreted the only difference between the male and a female aura is the vibration of Light each aura generates. In other words, the auras are non-sexual. They are neither male nor female. They are of a Light essence.

The fundamental physical difference between all embryos exists in the inherited combined chromosomes. The chromosomes merge to make the embryo develop into the aura's physical existence as either boy or girl.

The embryo's endocrine system's first task is if the embryo is male, it will release the male energies into the embryo to grow the male body. I call the male energies the 'conductor-based programmed energies.' If the endocrine system is female, it will release the female energies that I call the 'retentive-based programmed energies' into the embryo to make a female body. For this reason, I understand that it is the brain and the endocrine function that grows first to ensure they influence the remaining growth of the foetus with appropriate hormone releases. I understand that contained within the male-dominant conductor programme is the female retentive programme of energies. And contained within the female retentive programme of energies are the male conductor energies. There is a vast difference between the female retentive programme and the male conductor programmes. The male conductor programme is the fuel for powerful male hormones that constantly move in their purposeful existence to survive, dominate with strength, and procreate. The aura senses the conductor programme as a powerful force of strength.

The retentive programme is the fuel for the female endocrine system. It is not a replica of the powerful energy of the male. It is the peaceful and centred energies of much softer Light-infused hormones that are equally, if not more potent than the conductor programme. The female endocrine system is programmed and designed to be still, to hold and retain. It initially keeps the sperm of the male and the female's egg in the womb to grow into an embryo, and it will retain the baby in the womb until the baby is ready to be born. This retentive programme extends to the feelings of a woman. She automatically holds on to her feelings and emotions, her thoughts and memories.

The aura senses the retentive programme as subtle, soft, with magnetic sensations.

The conductor-based mind perspective mainly interprets this subtlety of energies as a weakness, female, vulnerable, or even undesirable.

The second function of either baby's endocrine system manifests when the conductor programmes release vast surges of adrenal hormones into the unborn body.

The aura of the unborn baby senses and feels the surge of power and the drive of the adrenal hormones as they stimulate and motivate the unborn baby to begin its birth journey within the womb. It is this force of adrenal hormones that will ultimately drive the baby through the birth canal. This journey will automatically determine and develop the blueprint of survival that imprints the newly awakened mind of the baby. The endocrine system continues its silent, invisible releases into the body throughout the child's life to pre-adolescent. The third significant visible influence of the endocrine function occurs when it triggers the body's adolescent hormone release.

In the **male**, the endocrine system triggers the conductor programme to release the sex hormones into the adolescent body. The power of hormone release, particularly testosterone, fires up a boy's body to rapidly grow and become the body of a man. His sexual awakening develops him physically into the shape of a man, and it also changes his voice into the deeper sound of a man's voice. It is a necessary change that completely alters his perception of himself and how he believes other people perceive him. From his new identity as a young man, he must also be conscious of his mental powerfulness that reflects his opinions as a young man. He must be encouraged to interpret his feelings into unique, individual, adult thoughts by developing the boundaries in his mind. In particular, the boundaries of respect, responsibility, and truth.

This young male may grow into his physical power and may display the acceptance of his expected role as a man. However, does his bravado perspective permit him to grow into an adult with the thoughtful individual awareness of a man? The strength interpreted by the young male's bravado perspective grows into thoughts of strength and power in his mind. His attitude drives him to want the independence that can inspire him to become a powerful, unique, strong young man. Alternatively, adolescence can be a fearful phase dreaded by the parents, which can be sensed and interpreted negatively within the boy's bravado perspective. He internalises this negativity within his mind, and it fuels his anxiety about his adolescence. This combined negativity adds conflict within the young man's thoughts. This conflict clashes with the beliefs of his family. In this conflict, he feels imprisoned, and he thinks his family are the jailers who hold the key.

The imprisoned mindset and the jailer mindset are the hero roles cultivated within the family dynamic of thinking. These learned and inherited roles automatically configure young men's minds to remain dependent on each other and their families. These young men always look outwards for others to meet their needs, fulfil wants, and find an identity.

Their parents do not recognise or know when they should direct these young males to look inwards and look into their unique hearts and minds to answer their questions. Physically, the young male grows into the image of a man.

Mentally, he may stay in the interdependent role cultivated by his parents within the perceived power of the automatic family dynamic of survival and bravado. The

potential of his higher self empowerment and its awareness remains invisible and unknown to him until he consciously seeks to engage it in later years as an adult. The
collective society also supports the containment of the
growing boy's mind within the family dynamic because
usually, the family dynamic reflects society's thinking.
This collective containment and control provide fuel to
the conflicted spinning within these young men's minds.

In their learned 'roles,' the boys tend to roam society in herds of lads. They find their identity, strength and
powerfulness reflected from the collective identity of the
herd-like minds of their friends and peers. Their mental
conflict reveals itself in their sometimes reckless, pained,
troubled bravado, and the young lads' wild behaviour patterns. As they grow into older teenagers, young men, and
middle-aged men, they continue to automatically seek
outside of themselves from their childlike bravado perspectives looking for the elusiveness of their perceived
entitled power.

In the **female**, her endocrine system triggers her retentive programme to release its hormones. The oestro-
gen and progesterone releases in her body begin her adolescence. These hormone releases are powerful and ignite the transition from a girl's body into the shape of a
woman. The physical changes to the girl's body manifest
and expand in the form of breasts, bellies, and bottoms.
Overnight, her mind senses the changes in her body, and
she begins to think differently about herself. She feels

the power of her sexuality as her attitude and behaviour towards boys changes. She intuitively feels she wants to attract, keep and draw a boy to her. These feelings of womanhood are the prompts of her intuition and endocrine system, stimulating her ovulation and the menstrual cycle in her body. It is an inspiring time for her, as potentially, her endocrine system is invisibly urging her to conceive and carry a baby. She doesn't understand this power within her.

Nevertheless, the invisible intuitive urgings are for her to find sperm to fertilise her eggs which her body is preparing to release. The girl isn't conscious of this silent hormonal process. She doesn't fully understand what is happening to her, either physically or intuitively.

The hormone releases manifest in her bravado mind as feelings of openness, isolation, loneliness, and heightened sensitivity, both emotionally and mentally. It all manifests in her body as feelings of excessive physical fullness, hunger, bloated belly, nervous exhaustion, tension, migraine headaches, or physical pain. During this time of change within herself, she becomes self-conscious. She is hypersensitive and is aware of her feelings. She is easily upset or hurt by other people's actions and reactions, particularly fathers, brothers and boys.

During this time, the young female should be encouraged to accept her body's function by resting herself when she feels sick. Instead, she seeks the support of the learned family dynamic of thinking. This perspective will logically diagnose her heightened sensitivities as her vulnerability and mental weakness. Plus, it will endeavour to control them with medication.

The medication reinforces her bravado mind and ensures that she remains strong and not weak, not suffering from the 'woman thing,' the sickness, or the moods. The ignorance or denials of her true feelings are acceptable to her inner mind's conductor-based perspective, reflecting the knowledge of women held in a male-dominant society. I believe the female is the conduit essence and intention of God. She is his plan for the evolution of the human race and the universe. She upholds God's purpose by creating the aura within the Light vibrations of her heart chakra.

The woman automatically oppresses this high purpose within herself. Her conductor-based inner mind is supported entirely by the structures of our powerful societies' collective conductor's dominant energies. The woman's oppression manifests as irritants and irritations, an exaggerated sense of fear, loneliness, and other anxieties in her conscious mind, but finds release in her automatic and unconscious body language.

The woman's learned mind keeps her conformed in what she thinks she must be and what she must be equal to in our male-dominant society. She relies on acceptable learned mothering abilities and her unique sexual powers of attraction to share and express herself, find love, and share love and compassion. Society continually tells and reminds the woman she is weak and vulnerable, that she cannot survive without the conditioned support of the power of the male. She feels it for herself, but she usually senses it more for the survival, protection and safety of her children, her siblings, and their children. She automatically spreads her heart to all these aspects of mothering, often without any need or recognition of her own needs.

Society diminishes the heart of a woman to secondary entitlement in the realities of the status quo. This entitlement breeds a lack of respect, a lack of honour, a lack of value for the woman, the wife, the mother. The patriarchal mindset sits in judgement of the female while she runs herself ragged to please and maintain a safe and secure home for her children.

Somewhere in her feelings of hopelessness and mental distress, she tries in vain to become more like the successful men in the status quo of our realities. She seeks the power and control of the male and the power and success of money. She, the empowered female of the Light of her heart chakra's purpose and intention, flips automatically into a void of powerlessness, a forced sense of survival by her male counterpart. By extension, she is shadowing her babies into the male-based bravado mind of subjugation in the search for man's power, away from their real purpose – Light and the evolution of Light. The female, who *r* *'s her dominant conductor mind, only becomes an* *' of strength, a replica of the male mindset.*

The question is whether the male must become his retentive influenced mindset so that the woman, in the reflection of the man, may once again become the role God designed and created for her. Does this duplicity within our humanity have severe consequences for the future of our civilisation? I believe it does.

I believe there are genuine differences between a man and a woman. We are not equal in the way society wants us to think we are. Our minds and our bodies have different purposes. The aura is the only similarity between the male and female. I believe the endocrine part of the brain is the power that influences the difference between the male-based mindset that is survival driven and the female mindset. Is the superior male-based bravado survival-driven perspective aligned with God's intention when He created the human being?

The Whole Mind

L et us revert to the image of the inside of the grape-fruit that helped me initially describe the contents of the mind. I use this image to help me assimilate all of this amassed information, and I have fitted it into the structure of the fruit that can be easily understood.

I focused on the membrane of the white pith that was the centre, an integral part of the fruit and seemed to be pivotal to the formation of the fruit. I took this membrane as the force of Light energy that is the supportive struc-ture of every cell of the mind. It is essential to the mind's existence and the aura, as the white pith is to the funda-mental support of the grapefruit.

The following aspects, segments and different layers of energies make up the whole mind.

The Layers of the Whole Mind

1. The invisible Light of both the aura and the chakra system of every individual also carries the indi-vidual Light.
2. The spiritual and religious powers inherited from within the family unit.
3. The awakened mind.

4. How does the newly awakened mind develop into the unique mind of the adult?
5. Aspects of the mind.
6. The invisible reflected Light of the suppressed aura.
7. The conscious voice of the bravado mind.
8. The automatic voice of bravado.
9. The 'we' voice.
10. Light consciousness.

1. The invisible Light of both the aura and the chakra system of every individual also carries the individual Light.

The invisible Light of both the aura and the chakra system of every individual also carries their unique Light existence of a higher God essence that I call the higher self. This Light is also the thread that connects every human being to their higher God essence. The Light transmits sensations of unconditional love that are available for each human being to sense and feel within themselves. The transmissions of unconditional love are subtle to our senses, and it does take time to understand and feel them. Humanity remains ignorant of the existence of Light because the mind spins in recognition of a powerful conditional religious and spiritual God.

2. The spiritual and religious powers inherited from within the family unit.

The bravado mind automatically inherits and accepts the reality of a conditioned God that exists externally to us, mainly in our churches. The religious and spiritual inheritance grows mentally as the unique and learned sacredness that exists in memories and emotions. The learned sacredness becomes the moral compass to direct each person to understand their moral code, right and wrong, not only in their mind, but also in society.

I have called this layer of the mind the spiritual legacy of religions. The inspirer of this layer of energy in the child mind is the child's mother. In society, the mother is the upholder of religion and religious beliefs. It is her voice that perpetuates the influences of religion. She is the person that freely brings her newborn baby to her religion, chapel, church, priest, and pastor. It is she who gives away her baby's mind and heart freely to these organisations.

The mother automatically bequeaths her religion to her child. Her baby inherits its faith from the mother. In Christianity, this is the ceremony of baptism. During the ceremony, adults are appointed godparents to speak on behalf of the baby. The chosen godparents accept the free will of the baby as their free will, and they swear in unison in the name of God to honour and obey Jesus and God and renounce the devil. The baby again loses its voice and free will to the powerful voices of other people. Because the mother directs this ritual, it is accepted entirely by everyone because society expects it. The mother, her family and society are united in their religious beliefs.

I have previously written of the commanding forces within society that created images of a god that people have accepted and absorbed into their mindsets that reflect the images of gods. The true purpose of these gods is to control and dominate the minds and the hearts of the various gods' congregations.

There are so many god identities arising from these religions. It is impossible to equate them all into any one single status of a higher force of unconditional love that should be enlightening for people. Generally, the forces of religions are interpreted in fear, pain, and suffering by their congregations. The religions flourish in wealth and power, control and dominance, poverty and famines mainly because these religions go hand-in-hand with the governments corrupted by greed and manipulations, and they are controlled spiritually by their religions.

In my case, my religious beliefs became my identity in my inner mind. They became the invisible layers of spiritual influences that clouded my mind perspective, my vision of society, and myself that forced me to believe in the existence of a conditioned God and to trust in a conditioned love rather than trust and believe in myself.

As a growing child, I followed the example of my mother automatically. How she believed in her religion, trusted in God, lived her life every day in religious compliance, her relationships, and her example of how she loved her children, husband, parents, siblings, and other people became the basis for my mind.

Following my mother's example, my religion kept me in an innocent, childlike, automatic trust, and belief that kept me relating to the different childlike images of God. I learned to believe in various powerful invisible spirits that could, at their wish, intervene on my behalf with Jesus or God. They are the hierarchy of angels and saints, and the deity opposite to the hierarchy of demons and devils.

The learned acceptance of religion and the unquestioning of religious beliefs in people's minds end up holding adults in their childlike, innocent, unthinking minds. This, in turn, leads them to seek love and partners from this same unthinking mind perspective.

I believe each human being must question their internal beliefs to find their unique truth.

When you question the existence of your religious god, your answers will reveal the infinite God that is the invisible internal part of humanity. I believe it is this invisibility that transforms itself to the human mind as their Light essence. It is from the perspective of Light you find a Light consciousness.

3. The awakened mind.
The mind awakens into existence as the baby travels through the birth journey. The baby cries and breathes himself into an awareness of its physical body as it separates from the mother. The newly awakened mind spins and churns in the learning of isolation, in fear of darkness, the fear of the unknown, and the trauma that was its delivery journey. The baby's mind shapes itself to survive as it becomes the reality and identity of the baby.

4. How does the newly awakened mind develop into the unique mind of the adult?

In the male, his automatically sensed conductor-based mind perspective is to survive. He automatically cultivates his survival skills from his perceptions and learning, which grow into his bravado, powerful, fearless mindset and behaviour. It means his learned mind drives him to survive, to feel powerful, to be strong, to achieve, be successful, and not feel fear or weakness. This mindset permits him not to acknowledge his weaknesses which are the sensations of his sensed retentive inner mind which he automatically suppresses.

In the female, she senses her retentive-based mind perspective is also to survive. She will cultivate, develop, and expand the cells of her retentive mind instinctually from her sensed conductor-based inner mind. Her perceptions and her intuited survival skills expand her mind into her intuitive, sensitive, soft, caring, and loving survival energies. This sensitive mindset inspires her to engage with creative, caring, and supportive roles during her life. The female will suppress or deny a lot of the inner strengths in her conductor-based mind. The denial or the suppressed inner strength of her conductor-based inner mind can flip her mind automatically from the sensed influences of her sensed retentive-based energies into her sensed strength of conductor-based mind energies. If her mind flips, it will work automatically from her conductor-based energies of strength with a driving perspective of survival. In this instance, this woman becomes an imitation of the male, driving forward in her sensed conductor-based mind energies, automatically suppressing her retentive powers. This flip of her mind into her conductor-based mind causes conflict in her body as the retentive energies of her endocrine system are programmed to support her female body. The conductor-based energies are programmed to support the male body.

I believe each human being is unique and different from every other human being. People are not the same as other people. They may be similar, but they are uniquely different.

5. Aspects of the mind.
The Mother Aspect of the Bravado Mind

In a perfect world, the mind should radiate in the vibrations of Light. Ideally, each person should be sensing and feeling Light automatically as their birth right. Instead, as each baby is born, their Light existence is expunged or suppressed into darkness by the sensed dominant driving forces of the endocrine system. The darkened cells of the aura are crystallised into mind cells when the mind awakens during birth. The crystallisation of the cells into thoughts and emotions determines at which vibration the mind works.

The newly awakened mind of the baby is reinforced and soothed by the actions, reactions, responses, and behaviour of the mother towards her baby. The baby's interpretative ability fits within the sensory communication between mother and baby. This free flow of energies continues to be emitted by the mother and interpreted by the baby's senses after it is born. It cultivates, influences, and develops the baby's mind into a reflection of the mother's mind. It means the baby's wants and needs reflect what the mother thinks she knows are her baby's wants and needs. The mother's wants and needs become the baby's wants and needs. The baby's voice becomes the voice that the mother expects to hear from her baby. The baby's mind expands into both the learned and passive sensations that reflect the mother's mind.

It took me years of research to find, understand, and articulate the mother aspect of my mind. I had to recognise the sensed powerfulness that became my brashness as I grew into and out of adolescence. I had to recognise the automatically learned ability to love in my thoughts and feelings. I had to identify the automatic learned control that I recognised was a reactive reflex to my intuition, to my paranoid and irrational thoughts and emotions in my mind. I saw I had automatically interpreted her powerfulness, and I had assumed and accepted it as my power in my mind. I had automatically accepted her powerlessness. I had interpreted it as my powerlessness, my pain, my way.

I began by finding the bravado protectiveness in my thoughts. I saw I had innately taken my mother's protectiveness towards her children. I both imitated it and interpreted it as my protectiveness in my thoughts, in my automatic mind.

I began to recognise the many self-created thoughts and feelings in my mother's perspective that I was thinking, voicing or expressing as me, my voice, my thinking. I recognised that I had not just automatically taken on my mother's mindset, I had also automatically taken on the mother aspects of the minds of my older siblings, which added to the layers of mothering in my bravado mind.

I automatically created the collective mothering consciousness in my bravado thinking and behaviour. It revealed as my constant and relentless automatic need to mother, save, nurture, protect, and please all and sundry. I also began to understand and accept that these mother aspects created within my mind contained not just my mother's mind dynamic, but I had also inherited the past generations of her family dynamic of thinking. I also accepted that I had inherited her impressions, thoughts, interpretations, and feelings of my father's family dynamic.

These invisible layers of a mother's consciousness of protective and controlling energies were an essential part of my mind that became the invisible magnetic mental forces that automatically connected to the similar vibrations of the collective consciousness of society. I saw in my relationships that I connected to my male and female peers as I had connected to my mother's mind. It was through her mind that I connected to my father and any other males in my life.

My mind in this state of invisible pain and openness existed in states of defensive or protective barriers. I automatically cultivated barriers to protect myself from feeling this pain. I was ignorant of the need for personal boundaries. I had no idea of how self-confidence felt. I had no clue of what self-esteem meant in my mind. I had no idea I had a higher consciousness and a Light existence within my heart chakra.

The mother aspects of the mind must be peeled back and severed to enable a person to feel the uniqueness of the individual sensations of their Light. The mother aspects in my mind were the most difficult to find, recognise, identify, detach from, and release.

The Father Aspect of the Bravado Mind

The father aspects of my bravado mind were a big reveal to my mental perspective. When I began my spiritual healing journey, I became curious about everything to do with the mind. During these years, I assumed that the mind was created in male and female energies. The male energies represented the thoughts. The female energies represented the feelings and emotions.

Now I understand and accept that the mind initially forms from the aura existence. Therefore, the father's mind generates when he is just an embryo in the womb. Throughout the pregnancy, it is imprinted by the protective and survival skills initially sensed, interpreted, and transmitted by his mother, making his mind a female-influenced energy tool. His birth journey awakens his unique sensations to survive as he struggles to live.

His mind develops and expands. It relies heavily on its perceptions of power and strength, as well as the example and influence of his father's mind and behaviour. The perceived mental power and strength are built in his child mind as the many powerful survival aspects of his ego and his identity as he grows into adulthood. The child's imitation of its father is reinforced repeatedly by the mother's mindset as she encourages these developments in her child, as she automatically revels in her perceptions that her child is the perfect, strong child.

These father aspects of the child's mind are nurtured, supported, reinforced, and upheld by the mother and by the collective consciousness of the family unit of siblings, grandparents, aunts, uncles, cousins, neighbours, peers, friends, boyfriends and girlfriends, and society.

These powerful forces of survival energies are the tribal energy mass of the learned and intuited survival skills that pass into every generation by man. As with the mother aspects, the father aspects contain the inherited subconscious and unconscious mindsets of the father, the mindsets of his father, mother and their family dynamic of thought and behaviour.

The automatic acceptance of the patriarchal authoritative rule and control in the form of the laws and voice of society, religions, schools, colleges, universities, careers, employers, sports activities, social circles, neighbourhoods, and nationality reinforces the father aspects as the power of the mind.

I found this layer of energy relatively easy to recognise and reveal in my thinking and thoughts because it was the power-driven aspect of my mind. When I finally began to express my inner voice of Light awareness, I was able to peel away these layers of energy and cut them from my consciousness.

The Sub-Conscious Mind

I believe a man cannot create and build a conscious and sub-conscious mind based on the conductor-sensed energies without automatically creating an inner mind based on his retentive-sensed energies. I believe a woman cannot create and build a conscious and sub-conscious mind on the retentive-sensed energies without automatically creating an inner mind based on her powerful conductor-sensed energies. The hidden third reality in each person's mind is their unique Light reality within their heart chakra.

Unconscious Mind

The unconscious mind is the unknown. It is the invisible. It is the accumulation of the intuited learned, pained, and shadowed cells of the aura contained within the cells of the mind. The depth of the unconscious mind reflects the reach or the want for power and success in the conscious and subconscious minds. The human may not know of the existence of the unconscious mind, and that his conscious and subconscious minds are automatically powered, influenced, and driven by the irrational urges of that unconscious mind.

The unconscious mind is created unknowingly, invisibly, and automatically by both the conductor perspectives and the retentive perspectives.

The discarded, denied, unknown, and suppressed feelings are unvoiced. They accumulate to become the emotions that develop into the unconscious mind.

"Where does the unconscious mind exist?" I asked Light repeatedly as I obsessed with understanding it. I did not understand where it existed within the mind. I eventually permitted myself to interpret that the unexpressed feelings of the aura exist within the cells of the learned thoughts of the bravado mind. The bravado perspective automatically discards the sensory truth it feels because it believes in its misapprehension that the bravado mind is the all-powerful strong mind, therefore, it automatically suppresses or discards what it feels is its weakness.

The bravado mind perspective automatically flips its sensed weakness favouring the proven learned, knowledgeable actions and responses. The sensed feelings are never discarded but remain within the learned, knowledgeable thoughts.

The unconscious mind retains the discarded, the suppressed, the hidden, or the denied sensory feelings of the aura that unknowingly exist and reside invisibly in the bravado mind and manifests for a person as their conflicted thoughts, chronic pain, vulnerable feelings, and emotions. It also includes the overwhelming urges, irrational thoughts and emotions that arise mentally without warn-ing. The existence of the unconscious mind is instantly recognisable in anxious facial expressions, in sensed anx-ieties, and the defensive or unpredictable body reflexes and behaviour.

6. The invisible reflected Light of the suppressed aura.

The invisible reflected Light of the suppressed aura re-veals the different colours of the suppressed chakras. In meditation, people sometimes see flashes of the different colours of the chakras. Sometimes people see Light. The reflected Light of the heart chakra provides unconditional support and is the invisible membrane of Light protection for the shadowed cells of the bravado mind.

In my ignorance, I placed no value on my feelings, or in my inspired thoughts. In my ignorance, I thought that I dealt with the wrong or unwanted feelings, emotions and thoughts that I saw as my weaknesses when I denied them, dismissed them, pushed them away, or projected them onto other people as their weakness. In my igno-rance, I developed a life journey of the imitated shadows and the spirit shadows with no awareness, no insight into the need to seek the internal difference of who I was as a Light person.

Light encapsulates and holds these cells until the adult mind takes ownership and responsibility for the whole mind.

7. The conscious voice of the bravado mind.

The white pith, the inner part of the skin, is what I call the conscious voice, the expression of the individual voice of power.

My conscious voice is the voice of my identity. It is the voice of association that is unique to me, and it is the tool that separates me into my individuality and away from the collective voices of other people. However, it represents the many inner voices of the different learned aspects and segments of the subconscious. The powerful voice is what I choose to say, and more importantly, it is what I choose not to say. This voice is the calculated projection of my perceptions that ensures the influential approval of the external mindsets of our families, husbands, wives, friends, relatives, and society in general.

8. The automatic voice of bravado.

The bravado voice of automatic expression is the unthinking, unquestioning, learned voice from within the bravado mind. This automatic learned fearless voice of bravado could be the voice of automatic survival, the voice of automatic control, the voice of the automatic learned security, the learned automatic voice of holiness, and the learned automatic voice of the law-abiding attitudes. The bravado voice is supported and controlled by the family dynamic's powerful voice and the voice of the collective consciousness.

9. The 'we' voice.

The 'we' used by people who speak on behalf of the silent people and those who cannot speak up for themselves. These 'we' voices belong to politicians, the hierarchy of religions, the hierarchy of civil servants within the government, the army, the judicial system, and the hierarchy within families that speak on behalf of siblings. They always begin their manipulation by saying:

'We the people must...'

'We the government say...'

'The judicial system is the only autonomous voice of law and justice...'

'We speak the voice of God...'

'We speak on behalf of the silent people...'

'I speak for my family...'

10. The Light consciousness

The Light consciousness or the higher self exists within each person's heart chakra. The individual Light is the invisible direct connection into the universal Light of God. From this awareness of my unique Light existence, I began the evolutionary journey of my senses, and it is from this point of awareness, I will end my effort to evolve as Lucy.

It was my Light existence that I needed to seek, re-connect with, and re-engage with as I began to explore the darkness of my mind. Through the Light of my heart chakra, I found the inspiration to develop the grounding boundary that enabled me to start to stretch my energies free from the confines and restrictions of my bravado conditioned mind into my unique individual self-awareness of Light. I began to trust that my Light awareness was an actual existence within me. I began to seek Light intentionally, and I purposely began to express Light.

As my Light awareness grew and expanded, I began to gain self-confidence and self-esteem that reflected this inner Light awareness. The Light awareness did not miraculously engage my mind by dropping out of the skies. It did not appear to me in visions or come in any form of religious phenomena. My Light awareness was always within my heart chakra. I just needed to find my acceptance of it, align my intention to its engagement, and learn its language.

The clarity I achieved from Light helped me dig through the many layers of my mind dynamic of learned thoughts. In my acceptance of Light, I accepted the most beautiful gift my mother has given to me, which is my Light vibration, my higher self, my connection to the Light of God.

My Dedication to Light

I choose to dedicate my intention
To seek your presence within my heart chakra
I need to see you in your Light existence
So I can recognise your presence in my heart
I need to sense your Light vibration
So I can feel you within my awareness
So I can recognise your truth
The truth of Light
So that I can feel your truth in my voice as I voice my
truth.
I accept I must trust my intuition
So that I feel your strength and make it my strength
I must look into the darkness of my mind
Because I understand, I have hidden you there
I must ask for your courage, so I can make it my
courage,
So I can recognise I am not my emotions
And I am not my thoughts.
But to accept I am you, I must seek you
To feel your strength
When I am afraid,
When I am frightened
When I am angry

When I am frustrated,
I am dedicating my intention to Light as I light this
candle
To reflect the flame of Light in the absence of Light
Until I ignite my Light within.

Cycles of the Mind

I focused my senses outwards to engage with the universe. I interpreted that the universe and its planets are energy-based in a similar way to the Planet Earth. They vibrate in a continuous silent spinning movement, similar to the ebb and flow movement of our oceans and seas. I discovered these spins are very subtle, almost non-existent to the perception of the human mind. I needed to trust my senses to interpret them and accept what I was learning from my interpretations. I began to see that what I had previously accepted as the eternity of the universe revealed as my reflected unique unknown internal hidden universe within me, within my Light. I became aware that its energies are hugely instrumental in providing challenges to all human minds to aid healing and evolution. In my bravado, I was ignorant of these spins and cycles.

I was very conscious of the planets – such as the sun and the moon – because they directly impact our lives. The other planets have become the focus of the powerful countries as their governments continue to explore them. They target planets in the hope of taking control and colonising them, to use them for their purpose. On the whole, our societies remain ignorant of God's original intention for each planet He created. I have intuited that society's days of arrogant and ignorant passivity towards the universe is short-lived.

I understand that since God created the universe, some planets have combusted, and other planets have restarted new cycles. These cycles have begun to affect how all the planets are working, and they are triggering changes within the universe and within the human being's mindset, altering the human perspective.

I began my conscious observation of the universe in 2000, and even more so since 2012. I can see various changes have occurred in the different planet activities that altered the cycles of Planet Earth. The reset to different and new cycles has been occurring in almost all planets in our constellation. In turn, these are affecting the cycles and the orbits of Earth's energies. They also affect the mental cycles within the human mind. These new rotations of the planets bring on sudden and unforeseen events that cause new beginnings and rapid endings of situations and relationships. These revelations of change in the universal cycles provide a period of massive transition for every planet, every person, and every society. The changes are not occurring at the same time. If they did, we would all be swimming in the sea of the universe. The changes manifest in subtle, singular ways. They contribute to altering the energy balance within the Planet Earth, changing its direction to a new yet subtle course, in sync with other universal changes.

The currency of the new transition is the truth. The human being will seek and demand the truth. Truth must be the truth and not a version of the truth, a half-truth, a calculated truth, or a manipulative truth.

As we experience some of these changes through our weather extremes, we accept them as climate change. These changes are manifesting physically for us in our disruptive weather conditions. These include the forest fires, earthquakes, and tsunamis that have become regular occurrences, and the ice melting from the polar caps bringing more water into our seas and oceans. In Europe, we are experiencing the hottest days and the wettest winters ever recorded in recent years.

The energy changes are manifesting in individual's lives also. For example, Pisces the planet was on a specific orbit for thousands of years. It suddenly changed direction about seven years ago and began a new, utterly different cycle to its previous orbit.

If you are a Pisces person, you will have noticed the change in orbit the most. The Piscean mindset, the most psychic of all mind dynamics, was previously set within the narrow lenses of controlled thinking and daydreaming. The new cycle occurred for them within their mindsets invisibly without their input, choice, or decision-making. Around that time, I noticed the Piscean people were and some still are, in substantial internal crisis in their minds. They suddenly realised everything they thought they knew had changed. Their core existence altered to a whole new mind perspective overnight and manifested in broken relationships, new jobs, new homes, and new but different relationships.

To help a person understand how these invisible cycles of change work, I ask them to imagine they are confidently surfing the sea in an inner bay with the occasional wave to manoeuvre and survive. Suddenly the sea and the waves swell, the surfer spins out of control and finds himself going in a new direction that was bringing him out to sea. The new direction forces him to surf the open sea full of new challenges. He is not just coping with small waves – he has a turbulent sea with large waves to navigate for survival. He is also dealing with all the new and unknown challenges of an unfamiliar ocean never before seen or experienced by a Piscean person. This image explains the turbulence within the minds of the Piscean people's mental, emotional and spiritual challenges.

I understand that in the past, Piscean people have perceived life through a long narrow lens. It meant they saw what they wanted to see and overlooked much of what they deemed unnecessary for them to see in their lives. Their mind lens has had to broaden with its new energy cycle. The old lens has almost disappeared, making their past lives surreal in their minds and the future uncertain and strange.

In this new energy cycle, they try to re-build mindsets, new identities, new careers, and relationships. All these changes provided by the universe help the human being change, heal, and evolve.

When I began to attend spiritual healing courses, my mentor regularly challenged us to think seriously about the different cycles of the universe that affected the mind.

In particular, he often spoke about the impact of Saturn's ruling planet, its rotations and cycles. I heard the Saturn cycle occurs every thirty years. I should have been listening and taking notes on my spiritual healing course. Instead, I was doing arithmetic, trying to make sense of the Saturn cycle.

The biggest revelation from my sums was that I was forty-seven years old at the time. I deducted a thirty-year Saturn cycle from my forty-seven years to when I was seventeen. I was seventeen years old when my father abandoned me in his unique and reckless way into the isolation of the world. It forced me to become an independent working adult instead of a student, daughter, and family member.

Even though I wasn't fully aware of the depth of Saturn's cycle at that point in my life, I began observing my thoughts and feelings. I tried to tie in big feelings and emotions to the Saturn cycle. I became conscious of a pattern of fear emerging in my thoughts.

I had stayed in my marriage. Was it because I was frightened of the consequences of not being married? Was I afraid of being alone? Was I afraid of again experiencing the fear, isolation, loneliness, and rejection I had experienced when I had to leave my home as an unprepared young teenager?

I also knew wives who divorced their husbands were shunned in very subtle ways by society. As the months stretched into years, the question of my relationship regularly occupied my thoughts. Why am I staying in this relationship? Am I too frightened to leave? Intuitively, I knew I had to challenge this fear within me.

I began by asking big questions about my partner and our relationship. In my heart, I already had the answers, yet I was too frightened to accept them. When I heard my partner's answers, I knew I would have no options except to consider leaving and being on my own.

I began to intuit in my meditations that these cycles started for me not when I was born, but when my aura generated. My aura and every aura generates in Light. It means the Light aura is perfect and whole in every way representing Light itself and God's intention. I then realised that the astrology point at conception is as essential to understanding my adult mind as the astrology point when the mind awakens at birth. For example, I was born an Aquarian, but when I worked the astrology chart backwards to find a conception point, I am a Gemini.

This revelation is general information because my parents are no longer with us. Nevertheless, this was a significant acceptance point for me in learning who I am. I saw the external influences that were determining who I was in my thinking and my interpreted feelings. My mind worked from an Aquarian-influenced perspective, but my uniquely interpreted inner perspective works under Gemini influences. My ex-husband was a Gemini.

My mother was Cancer, but her conception point must have been in Libra. The passive influences of these star signs drove me to a double passivity depth in my mind.

My son was born a Cancer. My father was Leo, but his conception point must have been in Scorpio. My daughter was born a Scorpio.

Throughout this revelation, I was mesmerised as to how little of me there was in my mind. I can see how the planets' influences are cycled and recycled until a person's mind understands the particular blocks that create their differences or obstacles in their thoughts and emotions.

My bravado-mind perspective carried the layers and layers of the unknown, secretive, passive, immaturity of my inner mind within its fearless dynamic. This passive immaturity knitted the tricky emotional and spiritual dynamics of my unique learned mind together.

I saw in my meditations that the first mental sensation registered in the baby's mind is one of survival that automatically triggers feelings of fear. Fear multiplies into its many existences within the survival drive. The physical pain of pushing through the birth canal radiates through the baby's body, triggering further sensations of fear. As the baby pushes, it loses its Light awareness to feelings of fear and an awareness of darkness. It also loses the comfort and safety it felt in the womb that flips it to feelings of loss, insecurity, and fear. When the baby is born and feels its physical self, the survival instincts continue to work, this time to remind the body to survive. The baby automatically breathes to survive. The power of living supports the awakening of the mind into a sensed, instinctual, survival mind basis that instantly crystallises the previously held sensations in the aura to thoughts and feelings. This then suppresses the aura and its layers of absorbed sensations to the inner mind automatically. It spins in a single vessel of an automatic existence, driven by the need to survive. The survival mind perspective denies its inner reality of pain in the suppressed aura. It automatically encapsulates all the energies of the baby's body as its unique energies, its unique power. The depth of the unknown pain in the suppressed inner mind determines the vibration the survival-based mind awakens. The suppressed inner mind continues to exist and expand to become the hidden invisible magnet of pained thinking and emotions that lay within all the survival thoughts.

I revealed these suppressed and hidden layers of my mind through the process of my self-healing. Although they were invisible and unknown to me, I discovered they are present in my adult mind daily as I become conscious and aware of my automatic fears of exclusion, abandonment, rejection, not being loved, and feeling lost. I also began to accept my irrational emotions of loss and fear that have been very influential throughout my life as they unknowingly influenced my mind in painful fears.

This insight into how the mind starts and builds as it spins is why I understand that it is not a blank canvas when a baby's mind activates at birth. It has already cultivated a shadowed internal mind perspective automatically. It is hidden and unknown to the baby and also to the baby's parents. In their ignorance of how their baby's mind works, the baby's parents will parent to ensure their baby survives, lives, and thrives. They begin to parent with what they think is the blank canvas of their baby's new mind. Their best intention is to parent well or even better than how their parents parented them.

Parents and society are also unaware of the higher Light existence within their baby, making the baby's mind different and unique. They are unaware of the birth trauma the baby holds within its mind that is unique only to their baby. The parents are ignorant of the movement of the baby's endocrine system that is continuing to pump the adrenaline-based hormones into the baby's body after the birth journey.

After the baby is physically born, does any adult tell the baby it has safely arrived in this world? That it has survived its first journey into darkness, its first experience of tough love, as it loses the comfort of the womb, the mother and Light?

Does any adult explain to the baby why we slap its bottom? Does any adult tell it why it feels so cold so quickly? Does any adult explain to the baby why it feels wet or hungry, or explains what hunger is, or why it feels so edgy? No, they do not.

Does anyone show the baby how to turn off the adrenaline pump within its body after birth? No, they do not.

Do we, the adults caring for this baby, understand that we are looking at the issues that will affect the baby's mind for life? No, we do not.

The observers of the birth do not appear to understand the flow and the power of adrenaline automatically generated by both the unborn baby and the mother to enable the birthing process.

How can we, the adults, help a baby stop the adrenaline pump release within its mind and body? How can we shift the baby's perception from its anxiety of being born to balance itself into vibrations of love and positivity?

I am afraid it is back to the mother and how she mothers and loves her baby. Yes, the expectant parents may well have read every book written on the care of both mother and baby. The mother is usually particularly diligent in this learning, however, the difficult, painful labour will trigger her unknown chronic pain. The massive hormone release into her body will also trigger the urge to survive in her mind. The drive to survive will evoke and reveal more emotions that she didn't know existed within her mind. During her labour, she will spin and spiral into different painful fears in her inner mind.

Along with the inevitable emotional and hormonal upheaval, she will also recognise an erratic, uncontrollable train of fearful thoughts running through her internal mind. These are all unexpected new experiences for her mind perspective to deal with. She will automatically revert to her learned and inherited survival instincts to begin to mother her baby. She hides or denies the emotions that she fluctuates in, yet they reveal themselves in her eyes and her words as her unspoken fears. These are substantial invisible challenges that she has not previous-ly experienced, but she must cope with them in a silent, internalised way in her mind. "This will pass," I often hear people say to a new mother when she cries her way through her 'blue' days. I smile because I understand it fades into memories until the mother herself is ready to release the experiences and transmute them into a Light awareness. In the mother's pretence to appear healthy, her automatic mind perspective gives an almost dismissive nod to her experiences of giving birth and becoming a new mother. She spins unknowingly in her bravado mind to become an automatically challenged mother full of her internal anxieties. It is from this perspective she mother's her new baby. It is from this mindset that the cycles are created and fuelled in her baby's mind.

The relationship between a mother and her baby is unique. I have endeavoured to articulate the vast general-isation of a mother's mind dynamic into three mindsets. However, all mindsets are peppered with influences.

(i) The powerful mother's mind bravado perspective reflects strength, success and knowledge, with a strict, no-nonsense attitude to the world towards herself and her baby. She nurtures her baby into physical and mental existence, with little insight into her baby's unique mindset.

(ii) The automatic mother is a mother whose mind is fear-based. She feels insecure. She mothers automatically and nurtures her baby through her automatic fear. Caring for and loving her baby as she experienced it from her mother, and as she remembers it. She nurtures her baby into physical and mental existence, with little insight into her baby's unique mindset.

(iii) The empowered mother's mind perspective nurtures her baby to understand its uniqueness, sensitivity, and individualism. She does this nurturing by encouraging her baby's mental and emotional development in a positive mindset of boundaries, developing independent thinking, self-confidence, and self-esteem.

The first two mindsets will rear their babies automatically. The baby becomes an automatic extension of the mother's mind and her life. These mindsets will carry the baby's need to sense and feel the power of an automatic adrenaline release within its dynamic. It means that their babies will endure the unknown side effect of this constant adrenaline release, revealing the intense anxiety and nervous tension in the body muscles.

The automatic, unknown need for adrenaline will manifest throughout the development of the child's mind. It can be the root cause of the mental problems that manifest in learning difficulties, as well as in physical and emotional difficulties, as the child advances into adolescence and adulthood.

The child of the third mindset will experience life from a straightforward awareness of the self. The mother will have taught her child the need for self-protection boundaries, nurturing self-confidence and self-esteem in her babies.

However, I believe every mother has it within her instincts to soothe her baby's survival mindset into a less intense reality. She has the power to recreate the sensations of unconditional love and to reset her baby's senses to feel the security and protection it felt in the womb and can feel again, but this time from the transmissions of unconditional love from the mother's heart. She needs to open her whole being to enfold her baby close to her, which will soothe her baby until it settles into its new, safer mind reality. The mother's effort will help the baby feel loved and find a peaceful acceptance of itself within its mind. It will bring balance to the turbulence of emotions after the birth journey.

This bonding between the mother and her new baby is not always encouraged by her medical support team or by the father of her baby, and as a result, the bond isn't always as tight as it should be. Regardless of which type of mother the baby experiences, the baby will automatically be nurtured in the learning of a survival existence.

How I understand the cycles of the mindset of a baby develops:

1. The First Cycle of the Mind

The first cycle of the mind begins with the generation of the aura at a Light vibration. The cycle of Saturn begins its influences at conception when the aura facilitates an embryo. The embryo grows into the baby that reflects the Light of its aura. During the birth journey, the baby's mind flips from its Light awareness and its high vibrations and drops into dense dark vibrations. This flip into the bravado reality starts the first seven-year cycle of a baby's mind. This learning journey will invisibly and unknowingly influence and determine every baby's mind perspective.

The next stage of this cycle happens when the child goes to school. The mother makes a big deal of her child going to school. It is understandable from a mother's perspective, but it does trigger the fears of the initial unknown layers of memories and emotions in the child's inner mind. The child may panic at the prospect of leaving the mother or leaving the familiarity of the home's safety and security. The fear or the panic sensed in the child's mind triggers the endocrine system to release adrenaline into the child's body. The adrenaline release triggers regression to the birth journey and its trauma in the baby's mind.

Going to school becomes a traumatic event for the mind of the child.

The invisible turbulence and conflict within the child's mind spin as the child struggles to cope alone in the classroom. These are known only to the child's mind perspective. It is a lonely and intense time for a child.

The child's invisible struggles to control the fluctuations within their mind can manifest physically in sickness with eyes, ears, noses, the respiratory and digestive systems.

How can this child be helped to grow in every way at school? I believe the teacher plays a pivotal role in the classroom. How each child interprets the teacher's face, the teacher's voice, and the teacher's body language is unique in each child's mind. More importantly, what the child does with the interpretation in his mind dynamic will determine how he learns and absorbs knowledge.

The child's interpretation of the children he sits with during class will determine whether he will feel safe with these children. How the child decides to survive the feelings he senses is equally essential. The child also interprets the general sensory atmosphere within the classroom, the schoolyard and within the school generally. The child automatically reacts either positively or negatively to the thoughts in his mind. This internal sensory interpretation in the child's memory can be very influential in whether the child feels safe and happy in school or whether he feels sad and unhappy.

The child's ability to interpret his teacher's dynamic and the classroom will build several more invisible layers of learning within the child's mental growth. If the child's interpretation of the teacher feels safe or happy to the child's senses, the child's mind's turbulence will recede. His teacher will have a positive input into the sensations of the child's mind.

The child's interpretation of the teacher may trigger a dislike or awkward feelings towards the teacher in the child's mind. Parents and teachers need to understand what the child does with this information in his mind.

These feelings can negatively influence his internal mind reality and can grow into fearful shadows. The shadows align automatically with the child's learned mental turbulence. Together they develop into feelings and emotions that are fearful, and they swirl internally in the child's mind making it difficult for the child to learn and concentrate. In these circumstances, the child becomes blinded and deaf to what his teacher is saying. The child's invisible state is sensory-based feelings that can grow into invisible emotions that automatically block the child's mind from absorbing and learning knowledge.

The process of education and the child's physical growth will automatically expand the child's learned mind dynamic. The parents assume the education of their child is a positive learning process. The learned mind dynamic of a child can be negative or positive perspectives supported by negative and positive influences. These are the mostly unknown influences that create and determine a child-mind perspective that will probably last for the adult child.

2. The Second Seven-Year Cycle Begins

At this time, the adults begin to demand responsibility and accountability from their child.

In particular, the child must learn, remember, and be able to verbalise their schoolwork. The child quickly learns consequences if the child does not know the answers to the teacher's questions. Both the parents and teacher push the child's mind to learn, memorise and internalise even more knowledge. They add to this pressure by then sitting the child down and testing their ability to remember and recall information. Learning and remembering are no longer fun for the child – learning and memorising can become a mental burden in the child's mind.

To further add to this mental pressure for a child, the brightest child competition begins. Parents and teachers now reveal the bright children, the talented children, the not-so-bright children and the not-so-talented children. The child sits in the sensory reality of knowing fundamental differences between him and the more intelligent, more talented children. Adding more pressure, the teacher and parents reveal the programme of physical activities. Who are the best runners, who are the best players, who are the best dancers, who are the best gymnasts? The sensory pain continues to expand in the child not asked to participate in team sports. The child not invited to participate in drama. The child not included in class groups because they look different from their pretty classmates? The child the drama teacher says no to because the child is too fat? Who is the child that is thrown out of music class because they are not musical? The child asked to leave choir practice because they don't have a singing voice?

How does a child interpret these sensory realities presented to them by adults on a minute-to-minute basis as they struggle through their school's teaching? How does a small child cope with the limited mindset and frustration of their teacher? During this second cycle of seven years, the child's mind will have learned to fit into the family dynamic of thinking, fit the teacher's mind and the class-room dynamic, and the school playground dynamic. The child's mind advances in the development of his learned thoughts. At the same time, his unique internal interpretation of feelings also develops. The child learns daily what is good, what is not good, what is right, what is acceptable and knows what feels right, what feels wrong. The child's mind learns from adults. The child's mind believes in adults. The child automatically learns behaviour from the example of how the adult behaves. It finds its strength by imitating the perceived power of adults. It also learns to interpret the silent unsaid mind of the family dynamic. It continues to expand its unique internal interpretation of feelings. The child's mind spins into its bravado learning and behaviour. The child's mind learns to please or dis-please adults.

The child's mind and the child's silent internal intui-tive interpreted learning combine to develop a mind per-spective that allows the child to make internal choices. These choices are not always clear for adults to see or understand, and they may not be the best choices for the child. The child finds the easy way in their inner mind. The child learns automatic responses, learns their me-chanical action and reaction. The adults' domineering need to coerce their child's mind to the adult's percep-tions of control becomes clear to their child as they de-mand to hear their child's instant answers, see immedi-ate obedience, and teach their child to believe in duty.

In the child's mind, it learns to defend itself. It learns to self-protect. It becomes angry, defensive, and even aggressive in thoughts and behaviour. It learns to survive, to resist the control of others. In other words, the child develops survival skills and how to cope with other people's authority by using its mind to build protective barriers. The unknown obstacles of self-protection grow to form a 'normal' mind existence into 'normal' thinking for the child. The child's perception defines its lack of choice or free will and will feel controlled by the adult. Even more critical to the child's mind is the child's understanding that the need to control and conform is more important to the adults than the child's feelings. The contained conformity automatically reinforces the silent frustrations and anger that fuel the mind of an adolescent.

3. The Third Seven-Year Cycle

However, towards the end of the second seven-year cycle and the beginning of the third seven-year cycle, generally about the age of fourteen, the child senses powerful feelings of change within its mind and body. It becomes aware of the glory in their adolescent development (refer to the chapter, *The Endocrine System*).

The adolescent mind spans the ranges from the power struggles of the growing knowledge of sexuality, the growing and expanding physical body, and the powerful expanding senses that diverts the child away from the limitations of its previous learning and conditioning of the family dynamic of thinking. If the child does not find its unique power from within the family dynamic, it will undoubtedly find its powerfulness from within its peers' mind dynamics. The adolescent mind is now running as the bravado self-determining, wilful self-governing power of force driven by the adolescent mind perspective.

4. The Fourth Seven-Year Cycle

The fourth cycle begins for the young adult when it reaches twenty-one years of age. I understand that it is during this the fourth seven-year cycle that the mind of the adolescent expands into the full-blown ego. It is a critical stage of development for a growing young adult. The ego may reflect the power of the family dynamic or their peers' power, where the young adult demands their learned rightful expected entitlements to life.

Alternatively, another person with a different ego may not reflect the power of society or the family dynamic, however, may instead reflect the powerlessness of the community, of their peers. This person may have developed an acute awareness of inferiority, non-acceptance, and isolation as his identity. This person's ego is alienated further from the approval of their family, community, or society by their actions and behaviour. The alienation deepens the sense of powerlessness within their minds, which drives this ego to engage powerful abuse substances to empower them and lessen their pain.

At this time, the real identities of grown children come to the forefront and manifest as the 'truth' of a person's mind. It is also on the fourth cycle's completion when the young adult is about twenty-eight years old that a new life cycle in their mind begins.

The Saturn cycle begins silently, invisibly, and unknowingly within their mind. The cycle of Saturn starts for a person on the anniversary of the date of their conception. Since very few of us know the moment of conception, we tend to work with our birth time. Therefore, the Saturn cycle's effects register in a person's awareness as they celebrate their physical birthday of twenty-nine years and onwards. The Saturn cycle is invisible, unknown, and becomes the automatic emotional prompter to the bravado's thinking. It works by revealing the person's unconscious, subconscious, or suppressed realities of their unknown, hidden mind's emotions and spiritual pain.

An example of this is when a person whose Saturn cycle has begun, experiences a conscious loss in some degree of vibration in their mind. The loss is tangible. The loss may be due to the person moving from their family home, losing a job, or losing their house. It may be from losing a parent, a sibling, a friend, or a relationship. The loss may be intuited and only becomes evident in the internal conscious thinking of a person who may recognise this lacking in their thoughts as negative feelings towards themselves. For example, the person may feel a lack of status not achieved as a loss of approval. A different person may recognise their fear of failure and it may feel like rejection or loss of acceptance. A person may recognise the lack of recognition for their achievements by their peers, bosses, or parents, which they may feel as a failure, a loss of status, even a sense of betrayal.

The conscious experience of loss for a person, should they explore it, should reveal the layers of the more profound losses buried, denied, or suppressed in the inner mind. The recognition of loss will reveal and enable a person to find their core existence, their central sensory suppressed mind dynamic and heal it. A person may find it very difficult to articulate these intense feelings within their learned mind. The learned mind knows how to be strong and not to feel weakness. Therefore, the learned reaction to feelings of loss is to escape it, to flee it. The learned action is to deny or suppress the feelings of loss and to pretend they are not happening. Instead, the mind's learned reaction will be to fill the voids of loss with something learned that is secure, safe, and acceptable to society. This automatic decision-making results in a learned solution by a learned mind to feeling a unique truth.

The obvious solutions are getting involved in a committed relationship, having babies, getting career-orientated, and focusing on ambition and success or buying property to amass security. These responses are expected and supported by family and society. However, each individual must eventually accept the reveal of their suppressed feelings and emotions. The universe and Saturn will continue to urge the recognition of the central sensory mind dynamic. An individual must engage the reflected opportunities that the synchronicity of the Light of the universe provides to help them accept both the existence and the reality of their sensory central mind dynamic. This acceptance of the need to find the true self and its uniqueness is the key to finding individuality. A person who finally accepts their enlightenment gift from the Light of the universe usually begins questioning and self-questioning everything within the individual mindset. From a new and higher mind perspective, the learned, projected self will reveal itself to a person who seeks it. The higher awareness also inspires the individual to apply boundaries like responsibility, respect, discipline, unique thinking, and personal spiritual accountability. This enlightenment gift provides the person with the opportunity to ignite and guide their central sensory mind dynamic back to a Light structure.

When I became aware that I needed to give my Saturn cycle my full attention, I was forty-seven years old. Looking back on that period of my life, I now see that I was on a very slow awakening to me, my inner self. My awakening was to the realisation that I was in a mental robotic stupor, living life at a superficial bravado existence. My awakening was also to the recognition that I had the massive potential to change my mind. I also realised that I could reconnect to my Light existence that was within my heart chakra. I began to accept responsibility for the consequences of my automatic past, my present thoughts, thinking and behaviour.

This reveal was the outcome of my Saturn cycle. It was a gift from the universe working for me, demanding me to become an adult with higher consciousness and an inspired mind perspective.

The Saturn cycle began its reveal in my thoughts, feelings, emotions, and dreams. The truth of my devastation when I lost my family at seventeen years old became evident to me during this time. It also revealed the reality of my broken heart when my mother died when I was twenty-three years old. I began to recognise the fear in all its disguises that was a constant influence in my mind, and it was crippling me. These revelations began a cycle of self-healing for me that continues to this day.

I can see in my bravado-mind where I automatically dealt with my Saturn cycle by ignoring or dismissing the revealing insights in my mind. An example of this is how I ignored or did not notice the old memories appearing in my mind relating to current events in my life. I saw I was repeating the automatic lack of decision-making in my past that controlled me in my present life. I saw the fear in every cell of my suppressed mind had automatically closed off many opportunities to change my mind dynamic. I was beginning to understand that I was accountable to myself for my life and my decisions. I also had started to look for accountability in my relationships.

I reflected on my life.

When I was twenty-nine years of age, I conceived my daughter. I remember I sailed through the pregnancy without any difficulty. I remember thinking this baby was not going to change me like babies changed other people. It was not until the end of my pregnancy that my high blood pressure levels meant I had to go to the hospital for an induced labour.

During my pregnancy, I remember telling the nurses and the doctor that I wanted a natural birth. I had practised a breathing technique to help me to control the pain of labour. However, in the induction ward, they began the preparation for my induced labour. I had no idea of what was about to happen. I still experience flutters of fear just thinking about my labour experiences.

The practice by the nurses at that time was to shave pubic hair. This routine involved a blunt razor and a cruel nurse. On top of the rough shave, they gave me an enema to flush out my bowel. I hadn't previously had an enema and was not expecting the force of release from my intestines. I seemed to sit on the toilet for hours. It was so harsh I ended up passing blood.

I remember lying slumped on the toilet floor, thinking that it was terrible. Now, I can see I felt weakened both physically and mentally before I ever started labour. I was in a haze of disorientation when a drip was attached to my arm. I remember my body went into one massive spasm of pain. I could not cope. In that spasm, I lost everything – my coping ability, control of the pain, control of my mind. The breathing technique that I had practised disappeared. I was spinning in a pain that I felt was wringing the life out of me. I remember screaming for help. No one seemed to listen. I screamed and pleaded for someone to come and hit me on the head, to kill me.

Eventually, they agreed to give me the epidural. The epidural gave me relief from the pain, but I now understand that it slowed down the birth. I can see myself lying in that bed, hooked up to monitors that checked the baby's heartbeat and my blood pressure. It seemed to take days before the baby was born. I remember a nurse coming back on duty from the previous day and talking down to me as I lay there. She said, "Are you still here?"

Eventually, my daughter was born. She was beautiful and healthy, and I began to breastfeed her.

I remember I had to stay put in bed for twelve hours because I had the epidural. I remember lying in bed feeling so small and so frightened. My sister came to see me. She said she thought I looked tiny in the bed. I was in horrific pain. The consultant cut me to help the baby be born. My episiotomy gave me five stitches that felt like fifty, and they were so tight and stiff and were so painful I seemed to cry in agony for weeks. I remember a nurse telling me the next day, "Get up and fetch your baby from the nursery." I said I couldn't get up that I was in agony. She said, "Stop feeling sorry for yourself and go fetch your baby now."

My husband was sitting on the chair beside the bed, listening to the conversation. He remained silent on the chair while I walked along to the nursery holding the wall along the corridor for support to fetch my baby for feeding. I still believe that the nurse's tone to me influenced my husband towards me at home. When I came home, I was still in excruciating pain. The weather was cold, it was snowing, and I felt cold. I felt my house was cold. I was fearful my baby would get cold, get sick and die. Everything seemed very difficult. My nipples began to crack and bleed. My daughter seemed to be always hungry, my husband seemed to be constantly hungry, and the dog always seemed hungry. It seemed like I hadn't dressed for weeks. I was in acute physical pain. I felt I had no one to care for me or believe me.

Now, I can see that I had been drowning within my mind in every way. I seemed to be over-anxious, frightened and fearful with my baby. I was frightened of the responsibility I knew was mine and nobody else's for the care and love of my baby. My body was not getting better. It still ached as the pain went up and down my spine. I didn't feel right. I didn't feel like me. I wasn't sleeping. I felt so frightened that I was not a natural mother, a proper mother. I felt fearful, lonely, and alone. I was feeling very sick. My stitches ensured that I could not sit or lie down to find any comfort. There was no one to tell me I was coping. There was no one to tell me this tough time would pass or that I was a good mother. There was no one to tell me my daughter was an excellent baby. I just saw all that was wrong.

Now, I can see I was very sick. I was paranoid about my baby. I often rushed to the doctor's office during the first two or three months. I did not understand that I was unsupported then.

I remember how my husband used to say to me as he pointed out friends, "Look at how so-and-so copes with their babies and children. Why can't you?" I would look at our friends and neighbours, and I would see happy and smiling faces, which triggered further loneliness.

I felt no better when I observed their mothers and their families surround them in what seemed to be caring, loving support. It seemed to me that our family was the baby and me. I could not verbalise or articulate how I felt. I was unable to bounce back to 'normal' me in my mind. I can remember one morning feeling so low and isolated that I felt unable to carry on. Over the previous days, I had often looked at the antidepressant tablets my doctor had given me and wondered how many I would have to take to die. One day I was not thinking of pills, but I thought I would jump into the river. I think my baby was about three months or so when I dressed her in her best clothes. I dressed, knowing I was heading for the river. I strapped her into her buggy. We headed into town to the river. It did not register with me that I passed over deep water when I crossed the canal bridge. I walked in an isolated, mentally focused state. I reached my chosen bridge. I stood looking down into the dark forces of the river, asking for courage from inside of me to jump. I looked at the baby. She was awake and looking up at me with complete trust. I looked down again at the water, its darkness and coldness. I instantly knew I could not jump. I knew I could not kill my baby.

As I walked home, I remember thinking it is not easy to die. A person needs a lot of courage to take the final step to die. That day I accepted that I was a fearful coward as I lacked the courage to die. That I was a 'weak person' appeared to be a reinforcing thought pattern in my mind.

I also knew there was no way out now for me except to live. Over the days that followed, something tiny seemed to change within my mind. On reflection of that morning's events, I believe the challenge in and to my mind to kill myself and my baby forced me to find a hidden strength to cope with my circumstances. I seemed to accept my situation. I relented to my new role as a mother. I made a couple of decisions that I would never go through this pain or feel so weak and vulnerable ever again. I reinforced these decisions by deciding never to have another baby. My thoughts lifted a little after I made these decisions. I began to cope better. My body began to heal, my baby grew more robust, and spring came.

I did not know that when I experienced and fluctuated in the high intensity of emotions and pain after the birth of my baby, that the unknown chronic pain of my birth journey with my mother was evoked in my mind. This chronic pain added further trauma to my traumatised mind at that time.

In my fifties, I found out the depth of those emotions relating to my new mother experiences. I can see that the trauma of the birth of my daughter unleashed the invisible mindset of my birth, including emotions of loneliness, aloneness, fear, isolation, sickness and fear of darkness buried within me. I discovered my feelings of fear, of not being wanted. During my life, I have been very conscious of my fear of being excluded by other people, not being wanted, or abandoned and left by my family and friends.

I now believe that when I faced the horror of jumping into the river to die and I decided not to jump but to live, I became consciously focused in my mind. I began to make decisions that helped me devise a coping mechanism to survive the distressing emotions I felt in my mind. I began to understand that making conscious decisions helped me control my feelings and emotions. I can also see after I failed in my intention to die that I had made another decision. I started to nurture my daughter by consciously loving her.

I was thirty years old when I conceived my son. I was thirty-one years when my son was born. He was my 'surprise' baby. He was my calm, joyful child that seemed to glow in love as I looked at him.

I remember when I accepted my pregnancy in my mind. I eventually went to my doctor. I told him I was in horror at the thought of the labour. He sent me to a different hospital to attend a different consultant. When I went to the consultant, I told him the horror of my previous labour and how terrified I was at the thought of the upcoming birth. I was petrified of getting depressed again.

In fairness to him, he reassured me that he would meet me and administer the epidural as soon as I went into labour.

He upheld his promise to me. My baby son was born. As he was delivered, massive fireworks went off in my head. It lasted for minutes. I said to the doctor that there were fireworks in my head. Someone said it must be something to do with the epidural. After the birth, I felt my steely determination not to breastfeed. The team left my baby son with me. I laid in rigid fear, refusing in my mind to breastfeed my baby because I remembered my previous breastfeeding trauma. To my deep shame now, I can say I let him cry until a nurse took him and fed him. I have felt so guilty about this, especially since I realised I could have healed my breastfeeding resistance with genuine compassion and support. The doctor cut me again to have this baby, though it seemed the stitches were less tight and less complicated. My body seemed to heal quicker.

Two days later, an earthquake happened in Dublin. I very clearly remember the nurse coming into the ward carrying a large teapot. She seemed to be frozen in the doorway as the hospital ward's framework shook for what seemed like minutes. She didn't panic. I cannot remember how I reacted. All I can recall is that image of the nurse. I had not experienced the tremors of an earthquake before.

I was home in no time bottle-feeding my new son without the horrors of my previous experience revisiting me. My babies thrived. However, I was bitterly disappointed when I discovered that the public health nurse that was supposedly supporting me after my son's birth was reporting our conversations during her visits directly to my husband unbeknownst to me. I felt disgusted with her. I could not look at her again. I often saw her out shopping or walking, and I was unable to acknowledge her. I felt so wounded by her deceitful behaviour. Why was the public health nurse belittling the trust between her and me? Why did she not understand how vital her visits were to me? Where was her courage to say no and direct him back to our doctor or me for answers? I will never understand this scenario that darkened me when I most needed compassion and support.

My Saturn return revealed as follows:

1. I was forty-six years old when I began to ask questions about my relationships.

I was in a similar mindset when I was sixteen years old.

2. I was forty-seven years old when I began spiritual healing courses.

At seventeen years old, I started a new life in the city.

3. I was forty-eight years old when I finally accepted my marriage was crumbling.

At eighteen years old, I was in full-time employment.

4. I was fifty-three years old when I finally left my family home.

At twenty-three years old, I buried my mother and met my husband.

5. I was fifty-seven years old when I fully accepted my spiritual journey was my life.

At twenty-seven years old, I married my husband.

6. I was sixty-one years old when my grandson was born.

At thirty-one years old, my son was born.

Since my sixtieth birthday, my healing journey has been profound, traumatic, dramatic, and powerful. I have been plagued with different flu-like viruses and sicknesses as I released vast, intense layers of suffering and pain buried in my thoughts and emotions. I am still dealing with revealing my hidden mind from the first three years I spent on this earth as a toddler. I have accepted this internal journey by letting go of the need to be powerful or successful. I now live in research mode as I continue to evolve, heal, and enlighten myself. I accept the deep healing my grandson is bringing forth within me. I am still on that journey.

What Is Mental Illness?

W hen I was growing up, and for most of my adult life, I was very conscious of the mind and mental illness. During my self-healing journey, mental illness and the fear of mental illness, in particular, were a huge hidden burden I discovered I carried automatically and unknowingly. This burden extended to all levels of my mind, automatically, consciously, subconsciously, and unconsciously. It also manifested in my physical body in bone and muscle pain.

From my current perspective of Light, I understand that this burden of fear was instrumental in containing my perspective in the lower dense, darker vibrations of pain within my mind.

When I was a young teenager, I remember hearing a conversation between my father and a neighbour while working with the hay on the farm. The gist of it was that they agreed that mental illness was part of our inherited genetics. I knew they spoke specifically of my siblings and me because they mentioned we had inherited this weakness from my mother's line. I pretended not to have heard them, and I kept working with the hay, but it hit me at my core. I felt the blow of it deep in my stomach. I could not believe that my father thought so little of us, his family. That he could think like this or that he felt he could speak to strangers about it, made it worse for me. The fact that he felt like this about his wife – my mother and his children was hurting me. I would return to it in my mind repeatedly. I often asked myself whether I had heard it right. Was it conceivable that I misunderstood that conversation as I never mentioned it to anyone else?

It was true. I revealed the grip of fear this conversation had on my mind. It had automatically influenced me negatively.

I further saw the energy ties that bound my perception of myself to that conversation and my father's thinking for most of my life. It fuelled high anxiety in my mind that I now know was influenced by my immature automatic acceptance of this conversation. I needed to unravel and transmute my anxiety before I found the words of that conversation that would unveil the initial blow of pain to my heart and solar plexus chakras. I recognised this fundamental fear was rooted in the basis of a lot of my automatic paranoid thinking. Fear was a huge block in my mind. A fear that was unknown to my bravado perspective fed my lack of confidence and self-esteem.

As my healing confidence expanded and I grew less fearful in my mind, I began to ask questions about mental illness. I recognised that mental illness was an umbrella term covering mental and emotional distress and unease within a person's mind. In my meditations, I lifted the umbrella to reveal the many different cloaks of painful static emotions hidden within my mind and unknown to my mental perspective. I saw I built automatic self-protection within my mind to protect me from mental illness. In my bravado mind, I refused to accept my weakness by automatically denying or suppressing my fears.

When I laid the contents of my bravado mind out on my desk, I began to understand how my mind worked. I saw my fearless bravado dynamic drove my mind perspective. I saw how it automatically reached for my learned power to feel strength in my mind. I associated power with strength – even when that power was dark and angry. In this perspective, I knew only power and strength, both mental and physical. I had little or no feelings because I automatically dismissed, suppressed, or denied them. I saw how I protected my weaknesses by automatically using any one of my mental barriers of power. From within my automatic protection barriers, I revealed a core fear of thinking that mental illness was my inevitable destiny. It was from this thinking that my hidden fears automatically grew and blossomed.

In my immature mind, I felt these weaknesses within me were unique to my family and me. I had interpreted within myself that this weakness was the link that would make me mentally ill. This flawed thinking started in my mind from a very young age. I continued to interpret and hide from the challenges I felt within the imprint of the father's aspect of my mind for most of my life. I had heard and accepted my father's opinion of my family and me.

I had automatically accepted his thinking as my thinking because I didn't challenge it for most of my life, not until I began my self-healing.

This dynamic within my mind permitted my bravado mind perspective to be judgemental and dismissive and carry an automatic disregard for weaker people. I can see that I was aware of compassion and charitable thoughts. I rarely showed this side of me. I judged and dismissed any sign of weakness, any sign of fear in my mind or the minds of people around me – very harshly at times.

Observation of my mind also revealed the vulnerability within me when I was required to show care. I played the role of carer, or I imitated the carer role from watching other people care. I was in my automatic learned role of caring, which left me pretty powerless when life challenged me to be an empathetic carer. Ironically, it was due to this struggle to make sense of my mind and emotions that my curiosity latched onto exploring the spiritual existence through meditation. It was my curiosity about the spirit that awakened some latent unknown me into becoming a spiritual healer. Back then, I was tinkering with the spirit world's potentials and possibilities when mental illness impacted ferociously in our family's life. I had many insights into the impact this pain had on my mind. However, the most interesting and revealing one was that I was terrified of it. I was terrified that I would become inflicted by it. I could not help or support the people in my family who needed me to be supportive and empathetic.

When my brother had a nervous breakdown, I found myself paralysed mentally, spiritually, and physically. I could not help him. I could not comfort him. I could not enable him out of his anxieties. I could not articulate that his emotions, which were mainly of anger, were not him. I could not tell him I loved him. I could not say a thing that was a comfort to him. I had no clarity of insight that could help him to feel stronger.

This insight about my mental vulnerabilities revealed my unknown terror of mental illness in my mind. My mind perspective could not control my anxiety about mental illness. It just spun into a mental paralysis, releasing emotions that flooded me in overwhelming fear. Time lapsed. The distance from my brother's illness helped me to look at my anxiety. I realised I had many different anxieties, not just the single anxiety of mental illness or the fear I could lose my sanity. I feared losing control. I feared being as vulnerable as my brother. I feared the power of the mental health doctors that left my brother traumatised further by their medication. I feared the power of the mental hospital that could keep me without my say so. I feared the power of the police that could cart me off to the hospital or prison without question. My anxiety-filled perspective had no adult insight about mental illness.

I realised that as long as I remained in my immature anxiety-driven perspective of mental illness, I would never heal my fear of mental illness. As long as my mind perspective remained that of a child, my mental attitude would remain lost in automatic focus and intention, floating in a melancholy state of unexplained pain. I realised my control mechanism that ensured I would not become mentally ill was also controlling other fears in my mind. The power to control my perspective and my anxiety-driven inner mind perspective were the two mindsets I had to release from my bravado mind.

I recognised I automatically created my emotions from my unexpressed and suppressed feelings. My sense of powerlessness, melancholy, fear, and sadness belonged to me. I had created them.

The fault or the blame I felt towards other people became irrelevant. It was my anxiety, my powerlessness, and my pain.

I saw my anxiety revealed, especially in my spiritual healing career. I was terrified of the spirit appearing to me either in meditation or in my healing. I sat for an extended period in my development classes, unable to accept inspirations or spiritual influences. My immature mind perspective refused to permit any inspired influence that challenged it because I had automatically associated the invisible spirit activities with schizophrenia and multiple personalities disorder in other people's minds.

I supported a lot of people during my meditation and healing careers. People always developed an interest in their empowerment through spirit and explored the different careers available to them through their spiritual development. People developed their psychic and their extrasensory awareness, especially in our meditation groups. I was always happy to support and enable this development. However, medium channelling was particularly sought after by people in our groups. People were interested in how it worked.

I discouraged medium channelling as I knew it required the transmission of dense, dark, powerful energies of spirit. From my experiences of sitting and facilitating meditation groups, I had witnessed these dense spirits refusing to detach from sitters' minds. I saw many sitters suffer huge mental upset and disempowerment by these spirits. For these reasons, I greatly discouraged the development of medium channelling. I saw in other groups when people did not engage their boundaries of protection. I was horrified at how open and vulnerable sitters were to the manipulation of visiting spirits. I thought the lack of personal boundaries and the low vibrations of the visiting spirits were dynamite to the sitting individuals' mindset that seemed to be unaware of the dangers, unaware that they needed protection for their vulnerabilities within their minds. They had no value at all on their fragile sanity. They seemed unaware of how easy the power of the invisible spirit can unbalance them.

Yet, people in my groups did not want to hear my opinions on medium development. I lost lots of people from my groups because of my stand on each sitter's necessity to understand the requirement of personal boundaries of protection and my insistence that each sitter should have an insight into their unique vulnerabilities before they welcome dense spirits to their inner awareness. People just wanted to experience the power of spirit and the sense of strength it gave them.

I have witnessed the way power-seeking spirit entities work. The spirits are not concerned about the person's identity or their wellness. These entities require power, any power to remain 'living.' These entities are not interested in a person's mental health or how balanced their sanity is. These spirits do not recognise evolution. They are interested only in continuing their one-dimensional existence of power. They are ruthless in their need to suck up energy that will power them. These spirits can infiltrate and influence a person's mind unbeknownst to a person's mental perspective. They are hugely influential in splintering the mind into different existences. Their different voices define the depth of mental suffering a person experiences when these spirits refuse to leave the mind.

My research into mental illness revealed the hesitation by the mentally sick person to consult a medical doctor. Their fear of the powerfulness of the doctor's actions and his numbing medications exacerbate their heightened feelings and emotions that are already flooding a terrified person's fearful mind. Another hesitation in getting a mental illness diagnosis is the bias and the attitude of smug powerful mindsets towards mental illness. They believe they are righteous in their 'saviour' minds to the perceived lesser, weaker, mentally sick people. Their religious-based thinking declares the superior opinions that distance them from weak or irrational people that may reflect on them by association. "Pull yourself together. You must be depressed," they say out loud in a smug voice as a solution to a problem, or, "Try to find a positive mental attitude."

An example is when a relationship breaks down, someone will always say, he or she has to be depressed or someone must have suffered from depression. My ex-husband used to tell me that he thought I lived in 'gubu land.' 'Gubu land' is the derogatory term he used to describe people's weakened or weaker minds.

Death triggers grieving, which is a form of depression. The weather, happiness, loss, and despair can all trigger depression. The trauma of my labour triggered my depression. I firmly believe my painful labour was not the reason I got depressed. Many factors contribute to the many types of mental illness. For example, addiction contributes to depression, schizophrenia, and psychosis. I understand that addiction is only ever a contributing factor to mental illness. It was essential for me to understand addiction is not the root cause of any mental illness because addiction is how the mind has learned to cope with chronic pain.

It seems the medical profession, without insight, continues to write its prescriptions using the same medications to dull, lessen, or cure people's chronic mental pain.

The single pill mentality does not heal, release, or free a person from their chronic mental pain. Through the healing of my mind dynamic, I recognised that my mind perspective automatically defaulted to pain and automatically created pain. In this reality of automatic suffering, I lacked any insight into me the person. I lacked insight into my mind. I lacked genuine confidence. I had no self-esteem.

During my weakest moments, when I felt the most vulnerable, I felt judged by people. I felt inadequate in their judgement. I saw their analysis of me in their eyes. I saw my weakness and my failure reflected in the eyes of my doctor, the public health nurse and my husband. Their unnecessary alienation of me just added to my burden of powerlessness that was already overwhelming me.

Another diagnosis of depression was offered to me in recent years when I told my then- doctor that I got up at about five in the morning to do my writing. He instantly said to me that this was a symptom of bipolar disease. This instant reactive diagnosis upset me. I had come in to tell him that I believed my cholesterol medication was causing me real distress, both mentally and physically. To ascertain how deep my distress was, he asked me about my daily living routines. If I had said I stayed in bed for most of the day, he would have said I was depressed. I feel he took the questioning of my medication prescribed by him as a personal attack on him, even a judgement or rejection of his expertise, and he needed to put me where he diagnosed me.

After a twenty-five year doctor-patient relationship, I finally relented to my intuition that it was over. I recognised that my relationship with my doctor was no different from my other relationships. I had placed my whole trust in his care of me without ever questioning him or questioning whether this care was best for me.

I finally stepped away and detached my mind perspective from the most profound, automatic, subservient, victim thinking. I no longer wanted to be dependent on medications. I trusted me, and I believed in Light that I would be ok. I knew I was fundamentally a healthy person, though I do have inherited high blood pressure. I now attend a compassionate doctor who treats me, and we find a medication that doesn't bloat or affect other organs in my body or disturb the balance of my mind.

As I began to trust in my Light awareness, I was able to diminish my irrational fear of mental illness. I accepted responsibility for my bravado mind, which I suppose, is my way of admitting that I was a little unbalanced in my bravado perspective of life. As I worked through and healed my issues, I recognised the pain in my hidden, unknown, unexpressed grief.

I found the pain at the loss of my mother, my marriage, my husband – the man I had loved, our business which we lost when it failed. I feel I also had to grieve the loss of my credibility that I had identified as me. I found I had no credibility after my divorce. It was non-existent and irrelevant to the status quo, but I had placed so much value in the worth of my credibility in my bravado mindset. I had relied on it as a wife, mother, daughter, sister, and friend.

There is no medicine created that could have addressed any of the pain-fuelled mental, emotional, or spiritual experiences I have had. I used the healing powers of Light to help me. I have trusted and accepted the inspired insights about myself, my mind, emotions, and my conformist, spiritual, victim thinking that enabled me to transmute these existences into Light.

My healing journey has revealed that the word 'depression' covers many intensely personal, intuitive painful feelings and emotions.

I firmly understand that until we begin to treat and respect a person in their unique and individual depressed state, we will fail in any attempt to heal depression. Our attitudes, our judgements, our medications, and our treatments will drive people into further dependent depths of mental and emotional despair and the pattern of addiction.

The projections and the perceptions of others no longer have the power to affect my identity or my mindset. I have finally accepted that my mind, emotions, and spirit are the created dynamic of my own making. I am the only person equipped to attempt to change this mind dynamic.

Addiction

What Is Addiction?

The dictionary describes addiction as a habit, a compulsion, dependence, a need, an obsession, a craving, or an infatuation.

I believe the imprints of depression are created in the sensory body of a baby during the following stages of its gestation period in the womb and during the birth journey as it absorbs pain automatically.

- The generation of the aura in the highest Light vibration facilitates the conception of the baby.
- The influential imprints of the endocrine system in the cells of the baby's aura.
- The powerful imprint of the mother's aura and her whole mind creates an invisible yet potent shadowed imprint in the baby's aura.
- The awakening of the mind of the baby during its birth journey.

I understand that depression is the shadow of invisible sensory pain within the baby's mind that registers in the aura from conception.

Addiction is one of the automatic tools a baby learns from birth that helps the baby's mind cope with the sensed pain of depression.

I believe the mind awakens in darkness. How the parents nurture and love their baby teaches a baby's mind to accept this darkness. The parents cultivate habits and behaviour in their babies that influences how the baby's mind grows and flourishes. The baby's mind may flourish in positive feelings that help the baby feel normal and feel positive within its mind. The baby's mind may flourish in negative feelings that help the baby feel normal, however, this normal is a negative and inferior mindset based on pain.

Or a baby's mind can fluctuate in both positive and negative perspectives. All mindsets need to cope with the invisible mind. It is how a baby, a growing child, a young adult learns to cope and survive with the invisible learning within their mindset that decides their mind vibration. This journey an addict must retake and explore internally within their mind, will help heal their reliance on drugs or alcohol or any other abusive substances or behaviour. There are no short cuts, no quick fixes, and no medication to fix addiction. A person must intend to self-heal and develop the internal discipline that will permit this healing within the mind.

I feel that this is not just a description of addiction. It accurately describes life and life's strife that we engage in because of the learned way we perceive how we should live our lives. The moment we are born and decide to live is when we automatically begin to develop the mind dynamic of learning. This learning develops into a strategy for life or until the person decides to change it.

In this learning, children automatically follow their parents' example of how they deal with their pain, chronic pain, mental challenges, temper outbursts, racism, violence, and bigotry. Children observe parents' behaviour all the time and are continually interpreting it. To find their sense of strength and identity, children imitate their parents' thinking, actions, and behaviour. They will have watched their parents reach automatically for their food, their alcohol, their painkillers, their cigarettes, and their social drugs to cure and mute their pain. Children from a young age begin to smoke and drink automatically. It is usual for them to want to show off the learned imitated 'cool' confident behaviour of adults. Children drink because they think it is fun. They learn and perceive from both family and society that drinking is permitted, acceptable behaviour. It allows adults to be happy and enjoy party time. When children grow to become adults, they rarely change their drinking habits or reasons for drinking. Adults drink as they drank as young adolescences.

Adults use drugs as they used them as young adolescents. The adults' thinking remains the same as their child-self or until the adult changes it. There is an excellent line in a song from the film *Crazy Heart*. An alcoholic country singer describes the effects of his drinking, 'when it feels like I am flying, I am falling.' It tells the truth because most people think they are having a great time, they think they are flying when partying. Although, the truth in the real world of their feelings and emotions is they are falling further into lower vibrations of pain and spirit. They are subjecting their inner, core feelings to more torture.

Addiction is not just to drink or drugs. Addiction manifests in our minds in many different ways. For example, how I thought I should love my husband and be a wife formed an addiction in my mind. People's relationships are addictive because they become co-dependent on each other. People can become addicted to their families because their relationships are interdependent.

People in these relationships cannot make individual decisions and rely on the stronger family voice that tells them what to do, reflecting 'normality' and acceptable behaviour. The dynamic of the family unit represents security for an adolescent seeking to become their independent self. Although fear from society and family is the block that stops growth. The teenager becomes addicted to this fear unconsciously. In the same way, people become addicted to religion automatically, without thinking or understanding their choices. In the learned addicted behaviour, people reach outwards and upward in their minds to their god-like idols for support and love. People become addicted to gambling in all its forms. People become addicted to their choice of sport –running, mountain climbing, or cycling. People become addicted to sexual gratification, violence, and pain.

Addicts seem to be unaware of their mental, emotional, and physical barriers and limitations. For example, they don't feel their loneliness, their psychological distress, or their physical sicknesses. They do not recognise the irrational emotional drive that fuels them in their need to reach for their next fix automatically. They seem to be only aware of their need to be high, to be at the party they have convinced themselves they are enjoying. Their failings do not mean they are not the cleverest of manipulators and the most cunning of people. Their abilities to emotionally blackmail and coerce their friends and relatives for their purposes are potent and compelling.

An addict has no hesitation in using and abusing people that love and care for them in the most hurtful, humiliating, and frustrating ways. An addict will deny and blame anyone and everyone without hesitation. An addict is also devoid of any sense of responsibility, particularly personal responsibility. For these reasons, an addict is a challenging person to relate to or maintain any positive relationship with. There is no other reality in their minds except their need to feed the want of their addiction.

I have interpreted and intuited that addiction grows automatically in a person's mind because the addict is ignorant of how his mind works. An addict believes their mindset is typical, natural thinking. They are unaware they are spinning automatically in the bravado of their learned mind that automatically denies hurt feelings and negative emotions that unknowingly influence or drive their pained powerlessness, isolation, and introverted mindsets. We cannot heal this void in their minds with medication. I understand through my awareness that we must only attempt to recover an addict's pain through the Light of their heart.

I learned not to automatically support an addict or any person in pain. I needed to support people unconditionally and consciously. I help a person if and when they seek to heal by supporting them while they turn their senses inwards to their inner mind and hearts to find the reasons for their disempowerment. It is from their higher perspective of Light and awareness a person begins their self-healing journey. The person or addict can reveal their unique mental dynamic or the reasons for their unique addiction. If an addict refuses to accept help to heal or perhaps may be too broken to think of an alternative existence, I feel they may be on a journey to an early death. Perhaps their journey is their purpose to living. This journey is equally as important as all the other journeys of humanity in the reality of God. I support the healing journey of an addict by transmitting Light vibrations unconditionally to their hearts.

Death

What Does Death Mean?

I believe each morning I wake up is another day's preparation in my awareness for the eventual death of me, Lucy Devine. I intend to heal and transmute as much of my mind as possible to Light before I die. For me, this intention means that I die as Lucy Devine. My awareness, my Light essence evolves into the higher vibrations of Light without bringing forward an ego or spiritual imprint of myself into the universe.

The idea of death and dying was frightening for me and continues to be for most people I meet. I discovered I carried this fear unknowingly, automatically within my mind for most of my life. It was equally as frightening to me as the prospect of death itself. I recognised that I was only conscious of physical death, in the sense that I could see how the body dies. In the main, I was unaware of what happens to a person's thoughts and feelings after death.

Back then, I believed in my religious God and His hierarchy of indoctrinations that told me what happened to my 'soul' when I die. I recognised that I carried another huge unknown fear of how God's judgment would impact me when I did die. I saw His pointed finger directing souls to enter the glorious realms of heaven to sit at His right-hand side. Or it pointed people to the damnation of hell and the subsequent fears of its paralysing fires and demons. I observed in my learned religion that prayers are full of egos and promises of spiritual bounty. The messages from these prayers tell us that the soul sleeps in death until it awakens on the last day of resurrection in the presence of Jesus Christ and God. I believe this religious conditioning is a myth.

On my evolutionary journey back to God, I have interpreted I will not find an imprint of humanity in the Light or God existence. I believe there are no egos, no deities, no queens, no kings, no hierarchy, no good, no bad, no pretty, no beautiful, no strong, no weak, no ugly, no good looking, no stupid, no intelligent, no rich, no poor. There is only the existence of Light and the reality of a higher God existence and an endless abundance of compassion and love for those who need it.

Light influences helped me change my entire religion-based thought dynamic on death, which erupted and crashed within my thinking after I began to build new insights about death from my experiences in my meditations.

When I started to sit in my mentor's rescue group, I was blown away by the integrity of the work performed. The group was attended by people dedicated to the rescue and healing of spirit entities. The people channelled spirit entities that needed to see a Light existence to heal and evolve from the pain of their current 'living' existence.

My mentor was the facilitator of the group for years. I had not heard the term 'rescue' concerning meditation, however, I soon became aware of the most eye-popping, jaw-dropping insights and revelations to death and dying. Initially, when I sat in this group, the energies that presented to the group challenged and frightened me. As I sat, I kept one eye opened. I knew I only dared to sit in the group because I trusted my mentor fully and entirely. Even though I had this trust in him, I lacked confidence and trust within myself. My internal fears always overshadowed my best intentions. I sat upright in rigid tension, waiting for one of the sitters to begin their work by channelling a spirit entity. I was fascinated and petrified at the same time. I now can see I was utterly ignorant of this invisible reality of the spirit world that I was privileged to be glimpsing and witnessing that gave me huge awareness into death and its invisible existence.

I was gripped with curiosity as I observed my mentor working. I was always mesmerised at his accuracy when he communicated with the visiting spirits. His questions to them opened their mind to accept the death of their body. He was so compassionate in explaining that spirit was not a physical body, but the image of a body existing in memory and emotion.

He never failed to inspire the spirit to believe his words and seek a Light within or around them. The Light further inspired the spirit to let go and release its shadows and pain.

From a new Light perspective, the spirit always saw a pathway open up to reveal family members and guides that waited to greet the spirit. Then they accompanied the spirit to the next part of its eternal journey.

Spirit never refused to move on from its earth experience, and it always released its pain, being content to evolve to a new awareness and a new destination in the spirit world. I was fascinated by my mentor's work ethic. His intuition and endless compassion for the sitter who channelled spirit in pain was god-like. The enormous healing work that occurred in this invisible world which we did not speak about was enlightening and humbling for me.

I understood that the group worked because the spirit entities were brought to the rescue group by their spirit guides. In other words, the group worked because it was God that determined the agenda for the evening. We, the group, did not sit there and evoke the spirit.

I understand these spirit entities are the individual mind aspects that did not transmute into the universal energy when their physical body died. I began to build my awareness and insights about what happens to the mind and the emotions when a person's body dies. I began to accept the invisible aspect of a person's memory can continue to 'live' on in the earth energies, in the image of their physical identity.

An example of this work began when one of the group's sitters channelled the spirit of a man who instantly said, "I am tired."

"Why are you tired?" asked my mentor of the spirit entity.

"I feel I have been walking for a very long time," he said.

"Why are you walking?" my mentor asked.

"I sell newspapers, but nobody seems to want them," he said.

My mentor asked what date was in the newspaper. The spirit instantly said, "December 1900."

Well, I was transfixed as I sat on my chair. I was speechless. My mouth dropped open in awe. I realised this work was an entirely new and different awareness to my previously learned experiences of death.

My mind was spinning with questions. The healing of this rescue was one of many that evening. I sat and listened, trying to absorb the insights of the evening. My mind gradually opened to the wonder of spirit and the amazing unconditional love of Light and God in their support of each person that dies.

In my naivety back then, I often asked why the Pope doesn't acknowledge this man's work and what he does for the dead? However, as he often replied to my many questions, "No one dies, Lucy, only the body dies. Knowledge cannot help these spirits. Awareness and the compassion of the existence of the Light of God is what make the difference. Not many want to find it," he often said to me in answers to my questions.

'I want to find it. I need to understand it fully,' I used to say to myself. I want to be able to help to do this excellent

122

and beautiful work. As I mumbled my words, I always saw myself sitting in my anxious state in meditation. I was unaware of the mammoth healing journey I would have to engage with before I could even begin thinking about doing this work.

Some years later, my mentor became ill. I voluntarily took up the role of facilitator in the centre. Three or four years into my facilitating career, I began a development group made up of people, mainly healers, looking to develop their spiritual awareness. As a group of people with similar high intentions, we needed to open our mind perspectives to Light's influence. We needed to build our unique knowledge of God's purpose for us as individuals, as a group of healers, and His purpose for the whole of humanity. I can now see that my Light awareness as a facilitator was not sufficiently enlightened to hold the group in Light. Because of this, none of us understood the high intention required to do this work, and the group fell away from its commitment to healing the invisible spirit. I learned I needed to evolve in my awareness. I needed to heal my fears within myself before I could begin to inspire people to become healers and facilitators, to seek and work in a Light consciousness. As human beings, we do not know our potential to live in the invisible existence, supported unconditionally by the Light of God.

During this time, I was also beginning to accept I could not communicate with dead people in the same way I interacted with living people. I needed to sense a deceased person's energy rather than to want to see or to talk to them as I had known them when they lived.

I needed to accept my sensory interpretation without hesitation. It was my sensory interpretation I needed to communicate when I was speaking to people about spirit, death, and dying. Sensory communication is the truth of Light, and it works through boundaries that keep relationships positive and empowered. I encourage people who are grieving to begin to sense their loved ones as Light beings. For example, attune to a loved one's senses by smelling their perfume or their favourite flowers, taste their favourite dishes they liked to cook or eat, sing their favourite songs, listen to their favourite music, or whistle a tune to them. It is important not to connect to them physically or mentally.

The sensory message of unconditional love works through a bereaved person's heart that connects to the heart of the person who has died. In the awareness of Light, the heart chakras can grow into the fullness of unconditional love that does not require a void of pain or any emotional or spiritual dependency.

I also needed to understand the unquestioning intrinsic automatic belief in the religious dynamic of death and dying. In my meditations, I asked Light for inspiration to understand if this strict belief system is related to when and how children connect to their religions.

I began to understand that when children learn to accept their religious god, they learn to accept the image of their god without question. Even if that image is a pained god, the child learns to obey and love the brutal, cruel, painful images, and accept the messages and rules from this god. The child's survival instinct automatically protects itself from its perceptions of pain. The self-protection barrier in the child's mind determines that the religious teachings develop to become the entrenched, pain-fuelled barriers that radiate the reality of the internal suffering god.

This pained, shadowed mindset in a child will always interpret pain, any pain, as love from their perceived injured mind perspective. This mindset does not change as the child grows into adulthood. It continues to understand, see, and project pain as a love that automatically prevents the mind from healing or growing positively. The mindset fuels the irrational, unknown fears that influence or overshadow any mental intelligence that may enhance the mind to grow or to seek any expansion in their learned mental perspective of their god.

If this is true, then it goes a long way to explaining our immature, irrational fear of the process of death, death itself, and the afterlife. Because adults perceive death from an automatic childlike perspective, there is little room within this thinking to question the invisible life or the living ego, its emotions and thoughts, or the existence of spirit. We have surrendered our responsibility for our minds and our journeys into the afterlife to our religious control. It is the religion's control that suffocates the intuition and curiosity of the mind required to question any god's existence and hierarchy and, by extension, question the ego.

I understand that when a person dies, whether it is peaceful or in distress, whether it is sudden or alone, the person never dies alone, but is fully supported by their invisible guides from the Light. Their wholeness as a person is automatically supported and protected by Light and the higher wisdom of God. The body's death completes after the aura and the third eye chakra detaches entirely from the body. The Light of the aura magnetises back to its connection in the Light of the universe. The whole mental structure of a person's invisibility is welcomed and guided into Light's compassion and supporting structures that ensure the easy transition between this world, Earth, and the universe. Unfortunately, as in this life, many mindsets believe they are stronger than God's will, or they disbelieve in any god's existence. They are self-determined in their mindsets and remain in their opinionated will to live, and as spirits, they attract similar consciousness within the universe. A Light guide will support this mindset until the person's free will decides to ask for help.

Similarly, there is the mindset of the person who refuses to die. It resists the potential to yield from the power of the mind and counter-power of the body. It is determined to live. The physical body of this mindset will die. The identity and mind perspective continue to survive, continue to exist in the invisibility of their thought-driven spiritual reality without knowing the body had died. This spirit mindset will continue to survive in the same powerful, domineering existence of their physical life and living. This mindset is no longer a human being, has no physical body, and exists only in the image and memory of a human being. It is invisible to the physical eye and the seeing eye of society. It exists in spirit only, and its existence is problematic. This type of spirit needs the power of the human body to exist. It needs to feel powerful, so it grazes for power in human minds. It preys on human vulnerabilities to sustain its reality of power and control. These existences continue to 'live' until they themselves ask for help to change.

I remember in one meditation where I observed an image of a farmer walking towards his cows. He patted and praised each one. The farmer then walked away from them only to return seconds later and repeat the ritual. I saw a Light figure beside him that glowed, but the farmer was not sensing the influences of Light. His only thought seemed to be whether his cows were ok. I sensed that he needed to ask for help to let go of this ritual. I became aware he wanted to change, and in that instant, he turned towards the Light figure and asked for help. His Light guide stayed with him as he took faltering steps towards an older woman shining in Light, holding out her arms to him. I sensed this farmer had begun another spiritual journey.

The obstacle an evolving spirit may encounter in the spirit world is its role identity. The person's identity before they die may release from them in the spirit world as they evolve into higher vibrations of Light. However, their relatives on Earth keep calling the spirits back to these past roles and them. In their grief and loss, they keep these identities as sacred in their minds and hearts, and they love them in the same learned automatic entitled way people have learned to love in their relationships. In the same learned way, people love their angels and guides automatically. People automatically transfer their pain and dependencies to them. People give up their power to them as they look up to them from their kneeling perspective. People unquestioningly believe them when they claim they come from God and accept them as God's special messengers without questioning their purpose, intent, vibration, authenticity, or credibility.

In the same conditioned way, people learn to suffer and sacrifice their pain and burdens in their sacrificial thinking, which help the souls in purgatory or the lost souls. The controlling religious influences driving these people's minds of suffering are upheld and acknowledged by their congregations as god-like, as God intended. However, this thinking leaves the individuals not understanding the implications of their irresponsible behaviour towards themselves and humanity in general. Humanity must begin to accept that a pained, conditioned, learned mindset cannot help another person, especially a person in pain. A worried mind cannot support a suffocating mind existence, a victim existence, or a spiritual existence of suffering. The shadows of the invisible realities continue to exist because the human being is determined to nurture them. The ego is reluctant to take and accept full responsibility for itself and its pain. Therefore, it is resistant to becoming an individual, responsible, adult person, and it remains dependent on the invisible angels and saints.

I realised that while I lived, I needed to transmute my mind and the emotions it contained back to Light. This insight clarified my purpose to heal and transform my automatic bravado mind into the wholeness of Light.

I began to see that as a conditioned learned society, we lack general respect towards the less worthy in our congregations. I am aware that the law-abiding, self-righteous people who feel so precious and confident of their connection to their god, automatically judge the people around them as lesser or wrong. That the righteous thinkers are no better than the alcoholic or the typical 'sinner' is the great truth for me. In God's eyes, I believe He seeks the truth and responsibility of the vibrations of the heart. God is not interested in hearing the human-made excuses that whine from the comfort zones of the automatic mind's rules and regulations. At the same time, we all remember the gospel when God tells us that there are many rooms in His mansion. God, in His wholeness, accepts all into His realm. The wholeness of God does not judge or reject. It accommodates us all in the different vibrations of the universe.

Some people think that we are all children in the eyes of God. I interpret this as meaning we are all children in our minds, hence our relationship with God is childlike. I believe a person cannot have a relationship with God without adopting an adult perspective. It is only through this perspective does humanity begin to evolve into the Light of their higher consciousness. Otherwise, humanity remains as children in their minds, existing in the different conditioned childlike vibrations within the Earth energies.

We all die – that is certain. In my enlightenment, I understand that death is not an instantaneous event or something that happens in ignorance. For example, the body does not just decide to stop functioning and die. There is a programme or a blueprint within each aura that determines the life force and its expiry. This programme is not a secret. It does not hide from a person's mind. It is readily available in all its answers – should the mind ask the questions.

From a Light awareness, I believe that the Light within, along with God's higher consciousness, decides the journey of a person's life. The blueprint for the future life journey exists in the wisdom of the aura. The distance the mind travels between the subtleties of the aura's intuitive awareness, the question of death and how the mind interpreted answers remains unknown to the bravado mind perspective. Instead, it automatically spins in fear and denial or into extremes of a survival drive that determines that the body must not expire. I understand that sometimes the idea of death registers in a dread-filled thought that turns into an automatic fear of disease and manifests in the body and provides the body with the opportunity to die.

It became vital for me to understand that each person's death is unique in their journey back to God. A person's decision to die must be respected by the surviving people, whether it is a conscious choice, a bravado choice, or an informed choice. We need to understand that death is an evolving process every individual must engage in, and there is so much more to it than the body dying. When we support a dying person, we are supporting their wish to expire and to stop living. It is not our purpose to override or disregard this decision. It is not our purpose to impose our fears and emotions on or in the dying person's mind.

The potential separation of loved ones by death is the pain we cannot bear to imagine. What we fear so dreadfully is the isolation, the aloneness that the surviving relative has to endure. However, instead of accepting this burden of grief and healing it, we tend to beg, plead, and urge the dying person not to die, but to stay alive to continue in their suffering so that the surviving relatives do not have to suffer.

Since I engaged in the evolving process, I have accepted death as just another potential in my life's journey.

I believe there is no day of judgement to greet me when I die. There are no pearly white gates that permit me to enter heaven. There are no lifts, stairs or tunnels to bring me to the depths of the burning flames of hell. I realise that if this is your belief, if this is your required existence from the universe, then God's compassion will provide that existence for you.

I believe what awaits me when I die is Light and my perception of freedom. I hope to feel free from my physical body's constraints and released from the burden of my mind. I will no longer exist as Lucy Devine. I believe different levels of awareness of me will evolve back into the appropriate vibrations of Light. The mind barriers or aspects of my mind I have not released will undertake a process of containment within similar vibrations of the universe.

The journey of death is an evolving process, whether that process is voluntary and conscious by the person, or in the involuntary, unconscious, or subconscious protraction of human thought. Evolution happens.

Evolution

What Is Evolution?

E volution cannot happen without the generation of the aura, conception, birth, living, and death of every human being.

When I write about evolution, I write mainly about my personal experiences of how Light awareness permitted me to recognise my pain that needed healing. I released and transmuted emotions, spirits and feelings to Light through my self-healing process. I lifted my mind's vibration from a pained existence to a pain-free Light-filled existence, which enabled me to see and feel a new reality of unconditional love. I hear you ask, "Why only the emotional and spiritual release? Why do you not speak of the evolution of the mind?" The mind does not evolve. It is a containment vessel that retains all memories, emotions, and spirit within itself. The survival instinct of the mind strives for power to ensure the physical body lives. It is this powerful mind perspective that ensures life and living continues even when the body dies.

The process of evolution through a Light perspective ensures the dismantling of the survival-based bravado mind, which needs releasing from all it has learned, its acquired knowledge, its drive to survive, and its need to feel powerful. Power or powerfulness do not heal or transmute.

Let me explain the physical and mental growth that everyone is so familiar with within their minds. During my lifetime, I can recognise man's mind has expanded hugely, purely by identifying the profound changes from the time I was born. The vast span of the intellectual achievements of man is recognisable and can be very quickly listed. I will start when I was born.

Our home had no electricity, water, or plumbing. Our farm relied on the physical power of my parents and the labour of hired men. In the early sixties, the government arranged to connect my family home and our community to the electricity grid for the first time. Our community members started to replace their horses with tractors and using milking machines instead of hand-milking their cows. My father was very reluctant to change or build on the farm. He remained in the mindset of previous generations. He did allow our house to be connected to electricity. Later he did buy a car and a TV. As the children grew, particularly my older sister, she replaced the hired man as labour. He only relented to buy the tractor and the milking machine as the older children left home. At that time, the superpower nations explored space and planned to send a man to the moon. There was a vast difference between people's everyday existences. I had lived without external influences like television, movies, or telephones until my early teenage years.

I can recall a summer's day when our family were out in the meadow, and an aeroplane flew high in the sky over us. It was such a rare phenomenon that we all stopped working to look up at it. I remember waving at it and wondering what it must be like to fly in an aeroplane.

As I currently sit in my own home, I can choose any entertainment that my internet connection will permit me to explore. My television provides viewing in abundance. I have a machine to wash dishes, others to wash and dry clothes. I have multiple choices of transport available to me. I have numerous food options available to me to cook, and I have various ways to cook. The temperatures within my home do not vary as heating methods and ways of retaining heat that were non-existent when I was born, have since been devised.

Society has made considerable advancements in technology, aviation, science, and space exploration. The brilliance of all aspects of medicine has altered the journey of the human being. Science has changed the conception process and how or when the body dies. They have advanced to replacing body parts and organs as they fail.

Most young people wear earphones they use to listen to their phones. They talk seemingly to themselves as they answer the phone that rings silently. In my early life, if you spoke openly to yourself, you were classed as mentally ill.

However, the mind remains ignorant of the existence of Light, the higher consciousness of humanity. It also remains unaware of man's real purpose, which in my opinion, is the evolution of the energies of man into the Light awareness of God and the universe. Therefore, man's mind remains mainly in survival mode that powerfully blocks any influences that may lift its vibrations.

The human journey of evolution begins with the aura's generation into a higher Light vibration than the mind, followed by conception, followed by the gestation period in the womb, followed by the birth journey. Deciding to live, learning to survive, and acquiring power become the remit of the bravado survival powerful mind. The invisible unknown in this journey is the generation of the aura into the higher Light vibrations than the mind. This ensures every human being evolves automatically without it knowing or understanding evolution.

Then there is the chosen life journey of Light awareness. This journey begins with the same process as the bravado journey. However, it changes and evolves to experience higher vibrations of Light by seeking the higher self, the Light within and the awareness of Light. Through the Light perspective, it engages free will, boundaries of Light through decisions of choice. The Light perspective permits the sensory journey into the mind, emotions, and spirit to release and transmute them.

I intuited that man created religion in all its aspects to explain the existence of God's invisibility to people. It developed God into the image of a human man. It created a human woman of purity that became impregnated by a spirit to explain the existence of emotions that occurred without the influence of or injecting the male sperm into the human body. It created the birth of baby Jesus to explain to people the birth of God into humanity.

I have previously written about my belief that Light was God, and it was my required destination in my meditations. I also told of my shock-horror reaction when I realised that Light is not the desired destination for the evolving man's intention. Light is a tool created by God that forms a scaffolding-type structure that helps every aspect of creation and the universe remain upright, supported while it journeys to evolve and align with God's intention.

As my Light perspective travelled through the different chakras and their retained conditioning, I began to see that man's journey on Earth is a deliberate invention by God. The life journey of man replicates in every way the downfall of the original aspects of God that fell and kept falling until they lost their awareness of their god's identity. Instead, they took on the emotions they were feeling as their identity as they fell into lower vibrations. They did not just create feelings and emotions, they created darkness. God created Light to support and hold them in their darkness. God also created man to be the tool that would actively release these emotions back to a god-reality.

My Bravado Mind

A s a child, I remember questioning the mind's existence. At the time, I was sitting at the bottom of the
table watching my father sit at the top of the table telling
us his family or talking at us or not talking at all, as often
happened when we all sat to eat meals. He seemed to have
answers to everyone's problems then. As I looked at him,
I clearly remember asking myself, 'Where is his mind?
Where does he keep all that he knows?' This question
time was silent as my father did not encourage discussion
or debate while at the table.

I didn't get any answers to my questions on those occasions. It was decades later, when I began my self-healing journey, that I found the courage to ask these same
questions, this time about myself and my mind. Over several years of meditation, I slowly gained sufficient insight
that helped me interpret and accept the answers to the
questions that had started to trickle into my awareness,
permitting me a glimpse at the different workings of my
mind.

During my initial meditations about the mind, I began
to observe and recognise the behaviour and thinking of
people close to me, those who influenced my thoughts
and thinking automatically, unknowingly. Looking back,

it appeared I was sponge-like in how I interpreted and absorbed those people's influences and opinions. This insight into my mind led me to question my understanding of personal boundaries. Did I know about boundaries, or did I automatically assume that my barriers were my boundaries?

I began to recognise then that my mind was not necessarily determined or created by my ability or inability to make decisions, work, or survive. I can see that it was running on several automatic spins, not requiring conscious choice from me.

I began to observe my automatic adult ability to interpret my everyday mental challenges in the same way that I had interpreted challenges as a small child when I learned to interpret and survive within my family dynamic. I realised that my interpretation from those very tender childhood years was pain-based and was repeatedly reinforced in my mind as I grew up. I also recognised that I connected automatically to the pain in other people's minds.

My learning in school was on this same painful negative sensory reality. I interpreted the books I read and the conversations I heard or overheard negatively against myself. I saw that my rigid religious teachings supported, influenced, and inspired me in this pain-based negative and immature thinking both against myself and other people. I recognised that this immature interpretation was unbeknownst to me because it was entirely normal thinking for me. I recognised I suppressed my feelings. Instead, I took on the perceived, conditioned knowledge of other people's opinions as my thoughts and thinking. In my mind, this ability to rely on other people's voices and opinions was the reason why my default to pain was so normal and natural for me. After many years of questioning how I had become so dependent on other people for mental strength, I found some clarity of thought that continues to reveal itself to this day.

During meditation, an image flashed into my awareness of myself as a small child sitting in the lower infants class while my older sister was in first class. At that time, the girls' national school had only two teaching rooms. My older sister and her class were in the row behind the infants. They always whispered answers to the teacher's questions and I repeated their answers aloud, for which the teacher praised me.

My teacher never recognised the prompts from behind me. I never understood as a child that I needed to learn my lessons and develop the ability to create my own unique answers. I got praised by my teacher for echoing the older children's answers. My sister and her class moved to the other classroom, and I became conscious of not knowing the answers. I also knew I had fallen behind the other children in my class, which was a continual source of embarrassment internally, as I knew I was not the bright child the teacher thought I was.

As an adult, a wife, a mother, I continued to rely on this sister's reassurance and approval to reinforce my mind.

Without question, I relied on her for my power. I never questioned her opinion. She was always right and never wrong. I never thought to source answers for myself. Even when I started to write, she was the person I turned to for direction and guidance. It was this same sister who told me I had no style in my writing. She told me her teenage son had a better writing style than I would ever have. I remember feeling devastated. I didn't understand what she meant about style, and she couldn't explain it to me.

I also recognised that this habit of automatically asking for people's opinions existed in all my relationships. I habitually relied on their views and answers to reinforce my mental strengths, which I can now see was a massive weakness in my mind. I can see that it was how my dependence on other people blossomed in my mind. I now recognise my immature bravado thinking was reliant and dependent on other people's similarly shadowed influences. Even though in my mind I thought and believed I was independent and strong, I know now I should have gone back to school to learn and study as soon as my children were in school, but my hatred for schools and teachers blocked me. The automatic learning block within me prevented me from maturing and developing. Up until I accepted this realisation, I had blamed others for my shortcomings.

Light awareness inspired me to detach from all influences.

I began to build a new sensory Light-filled reality. I believed and trusted I was cultivating a Light-filled mind interpreted from my higher perspective that did not rely on any of the previously learned knowledge and people's opinions that I had stored in my mind. Eventually, I realised I had difficulties separating my two mind perspectives. Even though I believed I was intentionally creating a new Light-inspired mind, Light showed me that I was interpreting Light and wisdom from my child perspective and not from my sensory awareness.

I was evaluating my efforts to work from a new perspective. I recognised that my lack of language, lack of understanding words, lack of education, and my internal fears put a massive burden on my senses and interpretative skills. It meant that I was automatically flipping my sensory awareness into the learning of my child-mind. I was shocked and frustrated to realise my child's perspective still entrapped me. To stop these influences and to detach from them, I stopped reading books and going to church. I stopped believing everything I heard in conversations. I stopped believing in people. I stopped seeking the opinion and the support of other people. This effort was tremendously difficult for my mind to execute. Sometimes it felt like the bones in my body were breaking as I painfully resisted the automatic urges by my mental barriers to regress, yet I persevered with my detachment process.

When I did regress, I saw that it was silent and automatic as I retreated to familiar ways to the comfort zones in automatically reaching out to others. It was an invisible conflict because my reach outwards to other people was so entrenched and embedded in my child-mind. It felt normal and natural to me because it was me.

I stopped seeking spiritual clarity from other people as I felt the spirit itself was negatively influencing me, both towards me and within me. I stopped searching for power in every way. I stopped engaging in pain with people, which was extremely difficult because seeking pain was my normal instinct.

My intention to build a new Light-inspired mind free of powerful influences did not evolve properly until recently, years after I began to release my pain and lift my mind's vibration. The fact that I knew how conditioned support and influence worked and how it crippled me mentally and emotionally, didn't mean I was able to instantly detach and apply Light boundaries to my learned mental barriers. The Light revealed my mind was so shackled and bound up in shadowed and conditioned influences that I needed to release it layer by layer, thought by thought, feeling and interpretation before I could begin to build new awareness.

I began to observe my inner mind from my new awareness, my perspective of Light.

Through my observations, I began to understand the automatic pattern of thoughts in my mind. For example,

I saw that external challenges evoked or triggered the repressed feelings that caused me pain. I recognised that my instant thought reactions to pain automatically triggered my immature, bravado learning into a domino effect of emotions that had me automatically responding to my pain in anger or fear.

I saw I rarely voiced my genuine thoughts or feelings. Instead, they spun around in my inner mind. They grew to become the irrational thoughts of conflict, doubt, frustration, fear, or anger which were corrosive to me, my self-esteem, and my self-confidence. The conflict manifested in my furrowed, angry face, controlling behaviour, and irrational emotional outbursts. I was mostly unaware of these realities within my mind. I did not question the challenges that triggered their existences.

I responded automatically in my dismissive behaviour without asking myself the reason, the why, or the how.

I reflected on what I had begun to recognise as the distance that existed within my mind between people and life itself. I saw how my self-made pained mental barriers secured the vacuum that fuelled this distance.

For example, I identified how I automatically and unwittingly interpreted my family dynamic's language into a mindset of fearful thoughts and emotions. I also interpreted outside influences from within my community that aligned with my family dynamic. A great example of this was how I interpreted the silence of the family dynamic and our community's silence.

My interpretations of the silences were intimidating and fearful for me. I remember as a child trying to avoid people because I felt their pain. If I could not avoid meeting these people, I would not look at their faces. I tried to avoid fights among other children. I avoided conflicts in our home by hiding. I avoided hearing pain by blocking my ears. Avoidance became an automatic learned barrier in my mind. These barriers continued to grow in my adult mind and blocked me from moving away from painful situations or making positive decisions for myself in my life.

My other interpretations of the silent violence were subtle and less physical, yet were nevertheless as effective as the apparent fears. The way a person nodded their head indicated anger towards me. A person's salute or if they shook their fist, projected their anger and triggered my fear.

The whispering of secrets that excluded me from confidences and friendships, the body language of rejection, the body language of superiority, the body language of knowledge – all enabled me to build automatic barriers of protection for myself because I took all of this personally, against me. The teachers placed their sticks for beating us in the classroom where we all saw them. They were personal weapons used against me. My father placing the horsewhip over the fire was his silent threat of the dire consequences should we misbehave. Above all, there were the 'cross' expressions on people's faces that instilled a fearful silence of avoidance in me. I recognised that I interpreted their 'cross' faces as their anger, and I avoided them. I interpreted all these people's emotional and mental limitations and baggage as my pain because I connected to them through my pained perspective.

I responded outwardly in a defiant, automatic manner in my bravado mind perspective. I saw that because I did not positively use my feelings to enhance my thoughts and thinking, my mind remained on automatic pilot, and that kept me underdeveloped and childlike in every way.

I recognised that I was unable to voice my inner feelings. My bravado reaction to this paralysis of expression manifested in many irrational automatic urges in my bravado mind. I became conscious of my feelings of powerlessness. I could burst into uncontrollable tears instantly if challenged. Equally, I could burst into angry responses that closed down communications with people. I recognised how I used angry words liberally and cursed furiously many times a day. I cursed at people automatically. As I dug deeper into my child-mind, I began to recognise the unknown anger that drove me automatically. I began to recognise the layers and layers of anger that I had automatically built to protect myself. I began to see that this anger had created the distance between me and life and people.

There were other barriers in my bravado mind that I began to observe. I recognised my habit of standing back in the shadows of my thoughts, dependent on my husband, following his lead in his views, actions and reactions or looking to my sisters, friends, or other people's lives for my mental direction. I recognised how I relied on my comfort zone of mothering to assuage my inner awkwardness with people. I can see that I cultivated a general caring aspect in my mind by developing my ability to mother and feed people, whether they needed it or not.

I recognised how people's opinions and comments closed my mind to my feelings. For example, when a friend would say, "You don't like that surely!" or "That hairstyle isn't nice on you." or "That dress does nothing for you!", or "You are not talking to him!" I would find myself doing what this friend or sister told me was the right or the nice one, or the prettiest option for me. When my sister said she saw a dress that would suit me, and I needed a dress, I would buy it without even trying it. Now I recognise I had complete trust in her and her opinions, yet I had no trust at all in myself or in my ability to make choices. I began to accept that my bravado perspective was driven automatically by the language of the collective knowledge, as it spun into and out of actions and reactions without it being conscious of my mind, its anger, passivity, evasiveness or avoidance, or its escapist thought patterns. I began to understand that this was the journey of my healing. I had to start travelling the hidden dark thought trails within my mind.

I needed to recognise and accept my ignorance about me and within me.

I can see that I did not identify support or the need for support in my life. This insight was ironic because I was cultivated and cultured in the support role within my family dynamic from my youngest years. I recognised my support role had become my identity and this learning was a significant ignorance which caused massive resistance, dependence, and reluctance within my mind. It meant that I automatically supported everyone in my life because it was an unquestioning action or reaction in my mind. It was me. I never recognised when I needed to be helped or supported in return. I did not understand the vulnerabilities within me that needed to be supported by a stronger person. Above all, I did not recognise the lack of support from other people's thinking and behaviour. I did not understand the necessity of sharing workloads or for sharing responsibility. I only knew one responsibility – my learning of collective responsibility, which I automatically applied in every part of my life.

I had interpreted and learned this sense of collective responsibility as a child. I continued to default to it in my adult life. From my Light awareness, I can see that back then, I felt supported when someone told me what to do. I can see that I automatically accepted 'orders' from other people. I saw my carrying out of these 'orders' as my way of being obedient, loyal, trustworthy, and fulfilling my duty so that life continued in an orderly, responsible way. I didn't recognise support, which meant for me that I did not value support. I can see how the lack of support during the tough times in my life forced me to pretend to be my learned 'strong' self and not express the weakness in my thinking, which was detrimental to my wellbeing.

From my Light awareness, I recognised my bravado perspective in its automatic assumption and acceptance of my strength did not see the lack of support in my life as a fault or a failing in others. Furthermore, my inability to ask for help was because I had automatically assumed that needing help was my weakness. This thinking formed my mind as everyday rational thoughts and thinking for me back then.

In the same breath, I can say that all through my life, I powerfully supported similar mindsets in other people. I can see that their entitlement to my mind and my automatic support became their strength automatically in their minds. I began to understand that they were the weak people as they automatically took from me, yet were unable to give me back support.

I began to understand that I needed to separate the difference between the supportive role and the adult version of me who was seeking to evolve. I needed to heal and release my inherited dynamic of thinking that cultivated and shaped my mind into the supporter role identity. This supportive automatic role that I thought was me, dogged me all my life. It fuelled my thinking that other people were more entitled, more important, more powerful, more worthy, which kept my thinking and behaviour lesser, even servile and in their shadows. I automatically assumed that I was an automatic follower of other people, the automated worker who was servant-like in my demeanour.

I recognised my thinking in my bravado mind perspective was a narrow, closed, conditioned, and pained mind that knew weakness and was frightened of it. My bravado perspective knew if the mind 'broke down' there were no medical answers, no ideas on how to repair it from doctors. While growing up, I saw the only solution was to lock the person in a mental institution and dose the person with medication. Alternatively, and even worse, these institutions were free to practice any of their horrendous 'therapies' to 'fix' a 'broken' person.

My bravado perspective saw that when the mental institutions diagnose their patients as 'cured,' they released them back into society after labelling them in boxes with a title for their illness. Those labels usually define them for the rest of their lives.

Along with this title, they are usually dosed with powerful psychotic drugs and told that their illness and prescribed treatment was their new reality, their regular lifestyle, their new identity. Society does not appear to understand that people can heal and grow from the mental or spiritual wounds they suffer. Instead, society throws away their potential to heal, to regain their mental health, and their ability to function as responsible and independent people by demanding they live their lives in their medically labelled, drug-induced 'fixed' states of existence.

Their drugged minds leave them unable to cope or function responsibly within society. When the medication fails to 'cure' the person, they are left for everyone to see as the broken one. Their community usually isolates them because of their extreme emotions and unpredictable behaviour.

From my self-healing perspective, I saw that my bravado thinking was profoundly wrong and insensitive. I needed to change my thinking, and I needed to accept that the mental fragility that I witnessed in other people mirrored the fragility inside of my mind.

I needed to accept that my mind was a self-created energy vessel made up of cells that reflected my feelings and thoughts. It was a shadowed, directionless instrument full of bravado recklessness. Depending on how I used my mind, it functioned more for other people's benefit than for my own benefit. I also needed to accept that I could heal my mind only through my Light awareness and not from any aspect of the learned bravado mind.

How did I create this vessel set in a dark tank of emotions and immature thoughts, a vessel that I used as a weapon or a tool at will? I saw that I had built a self-animated masterpiece of automated thinking, full of illusions, entitlements, and assumptions based on thoughts that had no depth because they were primarily other people's thoughts.

I now recognise clearly that my talent lay in my ability to interpret my everyday sensory world and turn this interpretation inwards to cloud my heart and my inner feelings.

I needed to change from this automatic default to pain. I needed to understand how I defaulted so quickly without being conscious of the regression. My intuition was on automatic alert, ready to instantly read every situation, every incident, every word, every look and behaviour that defaulted my thinking to my automatic learned pain.

My survival-based bravado perspective kept me living, breathing, thinking and feeling, although in a fear-stricken, pain-fuelled existence. I realised that I needed tremendous courage to accept the patterns of thoughts that had begun to unfold in my awareness. I prayed again for more courage to find acceptance as I realised that I created my pain, thoughts, feelings, and emotions.

I saw the necessity for me to begin to apply boundaries and detach from my bravado mind's pain. I also realised that I could only heal my mind by engaging my higher self, the Light within that permitted me to reveal my mind in a very safe and protected way.

Memories

When I began my mental inquisition, I interpreted that I needed to watch the entirety of my mind. I did not know how to do this at that time, so I began by focusing on my memories. I had to find out how I developed memories. How did I create them? Where did they begin? I needed to understand why they remained in my conscious thoughts. I needed to know why specific memories were so influential and lingered within my thoughts and feelings, determining my identity, sense of self, and behaviour.

A Memory Manifested

I saw myself as a young child, about eight or nine, playing hide and seek with my friends in the school toilets. I remember standing on the toilet seat and jumping up to look over the partition wall to find a friend in the other toilet cubicle. I missed my footing, and I fell into the 'dry' toilet. A dry toilet is a toilet seat covering a container that held the urine and excrement from all the girls in our school. I remember the smell. I felt I was dripping excrement and urine from every part of me in my memory, but I had fallen in feet first, so it must have filled my shoes and socks. I remember crying and crying. I vaguely remember my sister took my hand to lead me through the schoolyard to clean me with water from the tap outside the school grounds on the main road. At the time, I felt so dirty and so ashamed.

I began healing this memory, although my awareness of Light inspired me to require new compassion before it could begin. I intuited I needed to be patient and tolerant of my learned self. I needed to connect to my Light boundary of self-discipline to ensure I stayed in my Light awareness as I journeyed into my darkness and weakness.

It was an arduous process to begin engaging in my mind, as I had become aware in recent years of my bravado perspective that was unruly, intolerant, judgemental, impatient, and dismissive. I intuited that I had to work on the boundary of detachment in particular and other boundaries of Light before any work of healing and insight could begin on this memory. I detached it from my mind by placing a candle's flame between the memory and my memory bank. Eventually, I recognised that the memory was a child's memory, a child's perspective, a child's experience, but it oozed emotions that initially seemed new to my mind.

For weeks I continued to detach until I could no longer withstand the feelings flowing from it. One day I sat in meditation with my candle and asked Light for support and insight to heal my memory. I closed my eyes to focus inwards to attune to my Light within. After I sensed my sensations of Light, I grew aware of overwhelming feelings of shame. I became aware that I felt dirty in my person. I was also aware of feeling fear and humiliation.

I also saw the child-me within my awareness, as she recoiled inwards within herself when she saw the children of the schoolyard pointing and laughing at her as she passed them. I opened my eyes to come out of the healing. I felt awash with feelings and thoughts. It took a month or so before I realised that the memory and the emotions were still in my mind. I can now recognise that I had assumed that I had automatically healed the memory because I had revealed the feelings and the thinking of the child within me. I began to recognise the drift of emotions associated with my ability to automatically assume that I, the healer, the interpreter of Light, had thought I had healed. I assumed I was competent to recover this memory. "No," were the whispers I received when I questioned Light as to why I had not released the memory.

Light directed me to revisit the memory in meditation. I intuited that I needed to detach from the memory. I had to observe the memory. I needed to recognise what the memory told me, the aware adult. I saw that I reacted in two ways. I slipped into the memory's automatic learning, and I saw that I regressed to a child's perspective of myself in my mind. I recognised my thoughts, and I saw I was a dirty, shy, ashamed, awkward, and embarrassed child, terrified of what other people thought of me. I also observed I desperately needed them to like me. I saw that my learning from my memory had accumulated in other similar thoughts of inferiority I had automatically accepted as the truth about myself.

The emotions, however, were different. I felt the emotions of when this event happened were the same force of painful feelings I felt now as an adult. As an adult, I felt the violated child's emotions, the humiliated child, the shame-filled child, the angry child. Her automatic fear felt like panic to me. These feelings flowed upwards from my solar plexus into my heart and upper body, reddening my face in shame and embarrassment, shrivelling my mind, manifesting into awkward, throbbing anxiety in my chest.

I had not been conscious of these feelings as an adult, but I knew in my inner self that I had often felt shy, awkward, inadequate, defensive, and withdrawn as a growing child and young adult. I recognised that I was very easily embarrassed. I recalled the numerous occasions when I, the adult, wife and mother, witnessed myself retreat into darkness and the shadows of my passivity in my mind rather than face the external challenges from other people's emotions. From these shadows, I saw other people speak on my behalf or dismiss my presence. I also recognised that from these shadows, I watched other people appear to be freely enjoying their lives that seemed to me were without the encumbrances I felt within me. I saw how I automatically adapted my adult perspective to fit the shaped thinking of my child-mind that was fuelled by the invisible emotional influences within my mind perspective every moment of every day.

The following is an example of how I adapted my adult thinking to fit my learned child memory and the emotional and spiritual influences that were unknown to me.

I recognised the automatic reluctance and deep resistance I felt when my mentor asked me to become a facilitator in our centre. I saw how I recoiled within myself at the idea that I could sit in a circle of people, speak, and direct them about Spirit, Light, and God. I refused all opportunities to facilitate, even though I longed to become a facilitator in my mind. Plus, I was intuited by Light regularly in my meditations to become a facilitator to help me grow and expand my awareness within my healing channel. 'How did this happen?' I asked Light. 'How do I grasp what I need to do here to begin to release me from my imprisoned self?' I wrapped my memory, and its undercurrent of emotions in Light and I waited to feel inspired to accept the next level of healing.

A Memory Manifested

I have written in my previous book about my teeth and how they attracted and facilitated chronic pain throughout my life. I needed to find the source of the pain of this memory. When did it begin? Who started it? Why did it remain in such a heightened place in my consciousness? Why was it such an influence in my mind? Why was it such a raw wound that was me, my pain?

My memory revealed an incident from when I was about eight or nine years old. I had just begun to grow my adult teeth. I seemed to be unaware of my outgrowing teeth until one day when my mother sent me to the local shop for messages.

In conversation with another woman, the shopkeeper said that I was a lovely young thing only that my teeth ruined me, ruined the way I looked. The other woman looked at me and nodded in agreement. I left the shop mentally spinning in confusion and hurt. It registered with me that my teeth, which I had instantly become conscious of, suddenly became my ugliness.

I became aware of my teeth, and I became conscious of myself. I felt alone and isolated in my thinking about my teeth that stuck out. Soon in my mind, my teeth were the only reason other children did not like me. They were the only reason I didn't look or feel right in myself. They were my enemy. I saw how I felt anger when I saw people stare at me. I thought they were looking at my teeth. My teeth became the only reason that other children called me names. I felt my teeth were the reason these same children laughed at me.

I did not go home and tell my mother or anyone what I had just heard. I just wallowed in what the shopkeeper had said to me. I developed it into knowing that I was ugly in my inner mind from that day and for most of my life. My teeth were the radar point that permitted people's perspectives to effortlessly continue to fuel my invisible trauma. This woman, without intentional malice, began my conscious and my automatic non-acceptance of me by me. I remembered how it had been from that time I started to struggle in my thoughts. I became conscious of my inadequacies and my inner conflict about my imperfections in my mind.

As a child and adolescent, no adult ever questioned me about my teeth. The dentist didn't ask me if I liked them or if I wanted to change my teeth, nor did he volunteer any help with them. As a family, we only visited the dentist when we got a toothache.

Everyone assumed I was accepting of my teeth, but in my mind, I hated them. Imagine such conflict and heartache at such a tender age? And it could have been resolved so quickly by any of the adults in my life. This lack of care towards me by adults contributed hugely to building a defiance barrier in my mind as I grew and matured.

When I detached from this crippling memory, I recognised I carried deep automatic anger that fuelled a defiant, defensive, resistant mindset. I also carried within me an automatic acceptance of my ugliness and inferiority, which voided me of confidence as a child.

Even as an adult, I was drawn to dentists that were inadequate in that none of them could fix my teeth. I was angrily frustrated with them. I remember I went to Budapest with a friend to fix them when I was in my fifties. They took x-rays and photos of my then capped front teeth. They laughed at my hesitancy to accept their plan to fix my teeth. I sat in the chair seething in anger, unable to accurately compute what was going on in my mind, unable to understand my anger and frustration or why I felt the urge to run away. I ignored my inner urges and rather than waste the financial cost of the weekend, I reluctantly accepted their fix of my teeth, which was to insert a bridge in my mouth.

They proceeded with gusto to brutally extract my two teeth. It was excruciating and involved much suffering because their pain medication did not numb me sufficiently to control the pain. The language barrier was a problem because they did not understand that their pain medication was not working. Instead, they kept injecting me with the same medication as I squirmed in pain on the chair. I did not realise that this was a problem until the treatment was underway during the drilling and extraction. I felt brutalised and violated by the dentists. When I came home, I cried for days at the permanent loss of my teeth and the horrible feeling the bridge triggered in my mouth. I thought I would never get used to it. I completely regretted that I had permitted them to fix my teeth. This harrowing experience of foreign dentistry compounded my frustration and pain with my teeth and dentists.

It took me a further four years before toothache forced me to contact another dentist. During this lapse of time, I did not recognise that I was neglecting and destroying my other teeth. I didn't recognise the neglect of myself by myself. I could only feel the resistance and frustration towards dentists.

However, I have good news in that I have just completed a programme to insert dental implants in my mouth to replace the bridge this year (2018). I met two specialist dentists in Dublin.

Initially, I fought and argued with them. I blamed them for causing my pain. I saw myself resist their professional efforts to fix me as I sat for each of my appointments in my arrogance, anger, and fear. It took almost a year to fix my teeth. I cried to myself when I saw their result. My teeth looked perfect. I have asked myself repeatedly why I had not tried to sort my teeth sooner. Since I got my teeth fixed, many of the negative and invisible influences about my teeth have been revealed to me. I recognised how my face defaulted to the angry lines around my mouth that twisted my face in a protective and resistant expression. I recognised my default to anger in my mind when I observed people who seemed to only look at my teeth as we chatted.

I recognised that when I let go of these emotions, that pain flowed from behind them. The raw pain inflected almost sixty years previously was pumping hurt and injury through my whole body. My biggest revelation from this memory was my ability to neglect myself in a very self-righteous way.

I saw that I automatically thought I was protecting myself from pain. I had a childlike perspective of blame and pain. "Dentists are no good," I often ranted to myself and to anyone that would listen. "I hate dentists!" I often said. I felt every dentist I ever attended had failed me.

I recognised I had the exact same dismissive mechanism in my mind towards teachers. "You are useless!" I used to say to myself. I can now see that this was my father's thinking and his way of dismissing people. In expressing and accepting it was my way of coping with weakness both in me and other people without question.

A Memory Manifested

When I was about thirteen years old, I was changing schools. I overheard my father say to my mother I should not go to secondary school. "She hasn't the brains," he said to my mother. "She will marry in a few years; we will send her to the tech," he said. That was the end of the conversation about my education. The tech was a two-year college that provided practical courses to help prepare girls and boys for jobs that did not need the leaving certificate results required to attend university or college. It was the school of choice for me because my friends were going there. I knew I was not able for the study required in secondary school.

Over the years, I watched my older sister study for hours and hours without a break to sit her exams. I was also acutely aware that education was expensive, and I knew it was a substantial financial consideration for my parents. I knew they had to think of five other children when they thought about my school. I didn't care about my education, but I remember feeling so belittled by his opinion of me. I could only feel the pain of his insult. I was shocked and ashamed that my father thought so little of me. I could not believe that he thought I was stupid.

I now recognise their conversation did three things in my mind.

Firstly, my parents (my father in particular) indirectly hindered my education. I saw I acted out his perception of me. I acted stupidly. In my mind, his influences registered as factual, and I began to believe I was stupid. I already knew I was no good at learning, however, my father's words reinforced my inability to learn by vocalising his belief that I was stupid.

Secondly, my anxiety about my stupidity grew worse because my mother's silence meant she had not defended me or my 'brain,' which deepened my wounds.

Thirdly, I became ineffectual in my new school. I enjoyed it and had great fun. I learned to spoof, and I became a bit of a clown. Now I can see how I developed humour to mask my inner feelings of pain and inadequacy. I did not know then that I was angry.

Nevertheless, anger became the automatic weapon in my mind that I used against myself. The anger prevented me from learning and studying. My rage was a barrier to a self-fulfilling prophecy of justification, blame and irresponsibility.

I can see that in my mind, I was only conscious of how my father and mother thought of me, especially my father. I used to look at him and silently ask him, 'How can you think I am stupid?' I saw how many times a day

I called myself stupid when I failed in a chore. I felt inadequate when I was with my father. I also felt ashamed of myself around him.

I wrapped this memory in Light.

A Memory Manifested

My father was going to the local fair to sell some pigs. My mother told me my father wanted me to go with him. I was about ten or so, and I was excited and thrilled to be going. We started at about five o'clock in the morning.

Our transport was our horse, called Kit. The cart the horse pulled had sides attached to contain the load of pigs. My father had covered it with a tarpaulin to keep off the weather. The pigs snuggled up for warmth underneath. I stood beside my father at the front of the cart. He was driving the horse.

I had never been to the fair before. I had never been awake this early in the morning either. The cigarette that my father smoked provided the only light. He was telling me stories as we travelled to the village.

We were all familiar with the road, as we walked it twice a day, to and from school. My father had lived on the farm all his life and knew the road when it had been nothing more than a mud track. The horse was the most familiar with the road.

As we neared the village, we could hear other people's horses trot along in the same direction through the darkness. The fair held on the village green was a monthly event for the local farmers. When my father turned the horse into the fair that morning, the lights of the village green stunned me. I ducked down to hide with the pigs in darkness. I was not afraid of the pigs, though I was frightened by the brightness of the lights.

I sat peering out between the slats at the fair from my safe place. When my father found a place to set up his cart to sell his pigs, he took off the tarpaulin, and I had to adjust to the lights. I hopped out and began to follow him around the fair. I could hear and see the deal-making as farmers shouted prices at each other and spat on their hands before they shook them to seal their deals.

The shops and pubs were jammed full of people, mainly men. The animal waste was everywhere, even on the floors of the shops and pubs that were usually spotless, yet now they resembled the state of our farmyard. I accepted the farm's smells and dirt, but in school the village children mocked and taunted us, the children of farmers, because of this dirt.

I remember feeling confused between what I knew during the day in my school life and what I saw that morning. Daylight came, and the intensity of the dark early morning lessened for me. Once my father sold his pigs, we went home.

Two aspects of my mind became clear from this journey. As an adult, I can now see the shy, ashamed, and embarrassed child challenged by the scrutiny under the bright lights at the fair – frightened of being seen and embarrassed about who I was. Also, I could see I was familiar with the dark and not threatened by it at all. The adult me also saw how I automatically sought the familiar comfort of my hiding place of darkness in my life journey. In this state of shadowed comfort living, I was also avoiding accepting my responsibilities. I was unfamiliar with personal responsibility. It was from a state of this familiarity that I was automatically nurturing my children. What influences and conditions was I creating in their minds? I wrapped this memory in Light.

I am still seeking a resolution on how to clear these memories.

A Memory Manifested

I was in my first year in tech. My best friend, who I had met on our first day at primary school, got separated from me. We were put in different classes except for one or two subjects. Throughout the year, I noticed that our friendship began to expand to include other girls. I saw that my friend was becoming closer to another girl that had joined our friendship group. I tried very hard not to let my friend disappear from me, but she did not seem to notice me as much as before. I was getting cross in myself.

One day in English class, I pulled her chair from underneath her when she had to stand up to answer a question. She fell to the ground. I laughed, thinking it was funny. The joke I had intended for my friend turned on me – everyone seemed to laugh and point at me. That day I cried and cried in the school toilet and hid from my classes for the afternoon. My friend refused to talk to me.

A definite divide happened between us from then on. I was no longer an intimate part of our group. I was an outsider that sometimes tagged along with them. I didn't know a lot about what was happening with them. Sometimes I heard from other girls where they were going.

Now I can see all the emotions I was wallowing in at that time. I can see that I cared for my friend more than she cared for me. I can see that I was furious at being excluded by her and her new friend. I felt rejected by her. She had grown out of our relationship.

My hurt ached for a long time. As a result, our friendship did not last outside of school. We all separated. I lost touch with my school friends, particularly my friend from primary school, who was the most important person in my life at that time. All the feelings and emotions I felt during this time later revealed as the invisible pain-fuelled barriers in my thought patterns.

A Memory Manifested

I was about nine years old when I wanted to learn to play the fiddle. My father tried to teach me. The only time he could teach me was when he popped in to supervise my playing in between milking cows. No matter how hard I tried to play, I could not get it. One evening he shouted at me in frustration. "Give it up! You are useless," he said. I did give it up, and I accepted his opinion that I was useless wholeheartedly. I remember I felt the pain of his rejection deep inside of me. I stopped trying to learn to play the fiddle.

I did not show my hurt, yet I can remember that my sense of failure, my inadequacy seemed to make me work harder at pleasing him in other ways. It has taken me many years to discover that his instant dismissal of me had grown in my mind to become several of the self-created anger barriers in my bravado mind. I observed that I automatically and silently dismissed myself in my thoughts and feelings many times a day. I also observed that I automatically dismissed people in this same way. I observed the multiple learned thought patterns that revealed to me how I connected with other adults, particularly men, from this immature, hurt, defensive child perspective, constantly seeking their approval by ensuring I pleased them in some way. Mostly, I can see how I accepted their disrespect and dismissive behaviour towards me because it was normal behaviour in my mind. I did not recognise their slant of thinking or behaviour towards me, which I now know was abusive. I did not know how to identify the dilution of myself in my mind by other people. I did not know how to identify the dilution of myself by myself. I felt in my parental responsibilities that I needed to protect my children from this unknown emotional dilution. From this insight, I need to share three revelations in my awareness.

The first revelation I recognised was that my father's opinions of me were negative. His opinion of me that I was useless dogged me through my adult life.

Secondly, I can see that he had no real-time for me. He showed this by not organising my music lesson outside of his daily chore of milking the cows, which was one of the most critical jobs on the farm. This lack of adult nurturing and respectful interactions manifested in my relationship with my husband. I had automatically and blindly accepted I was not the priority in his mind and his behaviour reinforced this.

Thirdly, I recognised that my coping mechanism to hide my hurt was the self-imposed tool of working hard to please others. I had little time in my daily life to do anything except to think about work. I can see the child within me was still looking for approval from my father, who had died many years previously without ever validating me as his child or as an adult. I saw I was using the only way I had learned as a child to please my father, to automatically pacify my husband. I automatically and unconsciously worked endlessly, unquestioningly with and for my husband. I used to boast that I was the 'spare man' in our business because I could do any of the chores on the floor, usually if people were sick or absent from work. I can now see how I was trying to automatically please my husband and gain his love, recognition, appreciation, approval, and acceptance. He never asked for this enslaved attitude. He never felt he needed to validate me in any way. Many years on from this insight, I can say I needed my husband to validate me and to love me more than anything else in the world. He never understood my need, and so he never did.

Around this time, I intuited to look at the words that I used against myself in my mind that represented these negative emotions. For example, I studied the word stupid. I asked myself why I called myself stupid. Did I feel stupid, or did my mind accept I was a stupid person because authoritative people that should have known better told me I was stupid?

In my awareness, I reeled out the times I was called stupid or thick by adults. More importantly, I can see the regularity of when I heard I was a useless child. As a child, I accepted these opinions of me as accurate and as correct. I did not question them. I received them as my identity. When my awareness asked if I felt stupid, I accepted that I was not stupid and once again, I could feel the intensity of feelings, mainly of shame that I suppressed each time someone called me stupid.

I, the adult, was ashamed of myself. I constantly reinforced other people's opinions of me by calling myself stupid to please them. As an aware person, I must detach from this thought pattern and must not engage it again. I must seek to become a person who defaults to my Light awareness and not to the learned pain that was my past. I must seek to feel the wholeness of Light and accept this wholeness as me.

I found it easy to interpret this paragraph. I found it relatively easy to write it down, though I found it extremely difficult to practise this.

A Memory Manifested

When I was about thirteen or fourteen, I was at mass listening to the priest read from John's Gospel about love. It describes the love of a family, the love between the family members, the love God feels for each person. It felt beautiful, however, I knew I did not feel this love. I felt and recognised the absence of this love in my life.

A Memory Manifested

I was about seventeen years old. It was summertime. At the time, I was with my siblings picking stones from a field for my father. When my father returned to us a few hours later, he was unhappy with our progress. He gave out and was angry towards my older brother because he thought we had not picked all the stones. He was planning to re-seed the field. I thought what he said was unfair, and I said so. I answered him back and defended my brother. When I finished defending my brother, my father didn't respond to me at all except to say, "Get out. Get out this minute," as he pointed to the gate – the gate was the entrance to our farm. Whatever place in my mind I had found the strength to stand up to my father, it drained from me instantly. I went home to my mother and told her what had happened.

She said, "I suppose you can go to your sister in the city." Once again, she sided with my father.

It was not the brave or courageous me that left home that afternoon. The young girl who stepped on a train at seventeen was terrified, scared, spinning in an unreal reality.

I sat on a train, forced to work on a self-sufficiency plan in my immature mind to survive in my new life. I fought and argued with him in my mind as I sat on the speeding train. 'I'll never see him again,' I thought, 'I'll never go back home. I'll prove to him that I'm strong. He punished me unfairly, and for what? I always worked extremely hard for my father without ever being paid or asking him for money.' These thoughts spun around in my head. By the time I reached the city, I was angry, although I masked it with my excitement at meeting my sister and being in the city.

I learned a very harsh lesson in my mind that day. I learned I should keep my mouth shut. Forty years later and from my Light awareness perspective, I felt my anger as a wounded teenager. On identifying those feelings of rejection, rage, worthlessness and anger, I found the key to my self-healing journey. I found the glue that was keeping my memories and my emotions in place. My unknown, invisible, hidden, self-created anger was the backbone of my mind that was propping me upright. I needed to find this anger and where it hid in my mind. When did I begin to become an angry child? How did I not recognise my rage? I intuited to revert to my first memory and began to re-examine it to find answers.

From my new awareness of anger and how anger felt to me, I began to dissect the memory. I separated the layers. I took away the protective layer of thought that now felt to me like a shield of angry thoughts. I needed to look at each of these thoughts, find my contained feelings. As I released the anger, I became aware I was feeling fear and sadness. These were the core sensations that fuelled my inner mind.

During my meditations, I asked Light why I can't grasp the unfortunate sad girl within me for healing. I found there was no me. There was no girl that I could see to heal. There were sensations of fear and sadness. As an adult, I felt the loneliness, the bleakness of this fear and sadness that seemed to come from an endless void of darkness. I saw the need to detach from this void and surround it with Light. I still had not received specific answers on how to transmute memories.

I began to look at my dissected memory. I looked at the anger I felt, and I saw it was protective anger. I also recognised I carried internal anger built on my intuitive automatic sense of rage.

I observed my mind to find my rage. I saw how I seemed to rage about everything that seemed wrong to me automatically. I ranted about my experiences of unfairness, judgement, rejection and cruelty. I saw that all my rages accumulated into inner anger that was the great divider within me. I had the bravado external anger perspective, and I had the internal aspect of self-conflicted raging anger.

When I reflected on this anger in my mind, I glimpsed a big block wall that separated, not just the inner sad void, but all of the other voids I had interpreted as being me from the projected opinions of the outside world. On top of that wall, I was the bravado reckless me in my child-mind pretending to be strong and happy, pretending not to feel hurt, not to mind the name-calling and jeering that seemed a very natural part of my life.

I can see in my learned mind I became the name-caller, the joker, the teaser, the manipulator purely by my automatic acceptance of this behaviour and my inability to voice a difference of opinion. I was inspired to believe that I needed to detach from this revealing tapestry of bravado before I could begin to heal. I started to place Light between my Light perspective and my bravado learned mind.

I worked this detachment process for weeks before further clarity dawned within me.

Gradually, the shadowed faces began to manifest in my awareness. I started to reconcile the angry faces with the angry voices, which made up my dense automatic thinking. I began to see I was disappointed with my life. I was full of uneasy feelings and thoughts of worthlessness and powerlessness. These feelings had formed a protective, defensive, frustrated, reluctant, shy, and awkward bravado mindset. My bravado perspective submerged my mind's inner conflict, which manifested in my reluctance, and mostly in my inability to accept direction. I have recognised my angry hesitation that masked my invisible fear to accept or hear direction and influence from other people that could have helped and strengthened my mind. However, my immature angry protection kept me isolated in my thoughts, both from myself and others. Above all, I can see the lack of real intimacy in my adult relationships caused directly by the irrational emotions learned and developed from a child's perspective. I recognised other memories that contained emotions of shame, fear, anger, and embarrassment implanted in my mind by adults.

These emotions and memories formed part of the formidable wall of resistant barriers that merged with my defensiveness of anger and an inner reluctance in my adult mind.

Mind Barriers

What Are They? How Do I Create Them?

B efore I could move on to further, more in-depth exploration of my mind, I felt I had to recognise where my bravado perspective had hidden the tools of my mind. I began seeking these tools by acknowledging and engaging my free will, deciding my purpose, creating my intention, developing my internal focus, and speaking with my voice. I did not understand the necessity to exercise these tools that are uniquely me for most of my life. Since I began my self-healing journey, I recognise these tools are the implements of the Light of my aura that have enabled me to heal by attuning to and expanding my higher self the Light within.

Why did I suppress such an empowering part of my core self?

Why did my parents or my teachers not teach me the necessity to learn to make choices?

I was not encouraged to cultivate the importance of exercising my free will. I currently see the essential need for me and every person to understand boundaries and exercise free will. It is impossible to make unique decisions without exercising boundaries and using free will to respond to my mindset's internal and external challenges. I now call these essential decisions and choices my boundaries of Light.

My Light awareness showed me I had automatically buried my tools deep in my learned mind. I can see very clearly that I had cultivated pain barriers automatically in my mind when I should have engaged my boundaries.

My barriers were the mechanisms of various automatic painful thoughts and emotions that became the weaponry of defaults in my mind, defaults that I used to protect myself from my pain perceptions. I can see I instinctively and automatically activated my barriers in response to outside challenges.

I found that my barriers were the unknown mental magnets that automatically drew and attracted similar mindsets of familiarity. Their limited shadowed negative influences and their reverberations of invisible painful wounds overtook my core being. I recognised that my barriers manifested in many different aspects of my mind. For example, in my unfounded bravado confidence, I was right and not wrong in my thinking. I felt superior in my learned thoughts, in my automatic angry responses, in my automatic angry thoughts, irrational inferior thoughts, and emotions that churned my sacrificial mindset. In my smugness of unquestioned beliefs and behaviour, I recognised my irrational thoughts that contained irrational and fearful emotions that fuelled feelings of rejection, loss, separation, exclusion, abandonment, isolation, and aloneness – even the irrational fears of death.

This reveal showed me that I had automatically and unknowingly created my mind in the image of other people's opinions and their pain, which attracted me to people of similar thinking and thought vibrations. I was contained mentally within the reflection of my creation without understanding the consequences of the containment.

When I revealed the difference between my boundaries and my barriers, which was critical in the exposure of my mind's deception and avoidance, it enabled me to take a giant step in restructuring and expanding my Light awareness.

From my mind dynamic research, I discovered I had four main driving forces in my bravado mind that were upheld and supported by society's collective consciousness. These barriers developed systematically and automatically within my mind but were learned and resourced from the collective consciousness. They ensured the survival of both the mind and the body, and they cultivated my intuitive ability to mentally align my thinking within the collective control of corrosive power.

I have labelled these barrier shifts as my learned survival, my learned purpose, my learned containment, and my learned passivity. I began to look for these shifts of energy in my thought patterns. It became apparent that I had spent a significant part of my life sleepwalking in my mind.

I recognised I spent that sleeping period automatically fuelling emotions, particularly anger, to suppress my fears. I felt swamped in adrenaline. I was on a continuous spin in my mind, always thinking how to amass the power of collective knowledge, which was useless to me, and was of no support when I eventually woke up to my awareness. I became aware of the tsunami-like force of powerlessness, revealing itself to me as my unknown, invisible chronic pain.

From this perspective of sleep-walking, I had assumed that I knew the meaning of words and their application in language. This assumption of having the power of knowledge in my mind revealed a dogmatic mental barrier of superiority and a passive smugness in my mind perspective, which revealed significant mental blocks for me when I asked Light for support to change my mind.

I realised I had built my barriers with words formed from within this minimal intelligence in every aspect of my mind, in my thoughts and feelings, in the language I used, in my expression of words and my automatic thinking and behaviour.

With this insight into how my mind worked, I became the observer of my mind. I recognised and accepted it was an assumed, entitled, automatic knowledge-based power-driven mindset.

To detach fully from my assumed and entitled thoughts, I began to consciously check each word I used to make sure my words and language represented my intention to express the highest Light accurately.

I have listed the breakdown of words that I found were significant obstacles in my mind because I thought I understood them all. I assumed I knew them all, and I had an opinion on most of them. I thought I understood their purpose in the language I used. I discovered very painfully that I did not understand words or their meaning. In my ignorance, I had assumed I knew their meaning and their purpose. I realised that words have a purpose. I was ignorant of this purpose, of the energy contained within words and the engineered applications of words that make up a language. I found that my arrogance, ignorance, and irresponsibility within my mind permitted my barriers to automatically bury my Light uniqueness within the depth of my chronic pain and in my insecurities within the circumference of my childlike bravado mind.

I saw that I had assumed automatic learning of most words that I used, yet I recognised that I could not articulate my feelings into actual words when asked to express myself. I understood that I needed to apply the words to myself, to my existence, to my inner self, to express myself adequately and truthfully.

I saw that my intuitive understanding of words did not challenge or reflect my automatic thinking or my opinions. I saw my automatic assumption of knowing power buffered my mind in my automatic entitlement to life, my automatic control in my mind, and my automatic protectiveness in my mind.

When I looked to expand the meanings of words, I referenced the Collins Dictionary.

An example is for the meanings of the words *survive* and *survival*, I found continued existence, endurance, death. I found staying power, patience, stamina, security, safety, and grit. When I simplified these words further, I identified significant powerful aspects of my mind that had learned to survive regardless of the cost to my mind or my body.

When I applied these words and meanings to my inner mind, I saw the invisible shadowed emotions of fear, based mainly on fear of failure, fear of starvation, fear of death and darkness. When I released these emotions, I revealed feelings of loss and lost feelings of pain.

Similarly, when I looked to expand the meaning of *purpose*, I found reason, intention, drive, and ambition. When I simplified these words further, I identified principle, function, aim, objective, goal, determination, resolution, persistence, perseverance, indifference, and tenacity.

When I applied these meanings to my inner mind, I identified my lack of unique purpose. I saw I had adapted the family dynamic and society's automatic purpose as my force of mind. I recognised my automatic purpose enabled my powerlessness, my paralysis mentally and spiritually.

Similarly, when I looked to expand the meaning of *containment*, I found repression, suppression, control, restraint, inhibition, and expression. When I simplified this list, I found repression, oppression, subjugation, domination, authoritarianism, tyranny, despotism, and cruelty.

Oppression: domination, coercion, cruelty.

Subjugation: defeat, overthrow, conquest.

Control: manage, rule, and restrain, manipulation, influence, restraint, limitation, regulation.

Suppression: censorship, secrecy, conspiracies, dominance.

Restraint: self-control, limitation, captivity, protection.

Inhibition: reserve, hang-up, shyness, embarrassment, self-consciousness, reticence.

Expression: looks, appearance, phrase, illustration.

When I applied these meanings to my inner mind, I recognised the many aspects of my bravado mind that controlled me automatically in anger and resistance, however, kept me mentally immature in my child learning. When I released these thought patterns, I revealed an inner mind fuelled by fear of loss that contained inner based fears of rejection, inadequacy, and fear of failure.

Similarly, when I sought the meaning of *passivity*, I found obedience, tameness, submissiveness, humility, compliance and inaction.

Obedience: duty, deference, conformity, disobedience.

Tameness: gentleness, meekness, acceptance, peacefulness, docility.

Submissiveness: humbleness, timidity, modesty, mildness.

Compliance: fulfilment, obedience, agreement, resistance.

When I applied these meanings to my inner mind, I found the automatic passive aspects influenced by shadows and darkness that made up significant layers of my mind.

When I recognised passivity in my thoughts and feelings, I finally recognised my automatic acceptance and engagement of a learned conditioned love. I recognised my automatic assumption in my inner mind that my family loved me. I believed I was a loved person, and I assumed I loved people in return. I found my entitled and conditioned thoughts about love. I found my conditioned reasons to love. I found my childish ways to maintain love. I discovered my conditioned expressions of love. I found the hurt feelings that existed in a void of darkness because of my inability to love unconditionally.

I began to understand these words' energies and how I automatically connected to them through my perceptions. My perceptions based on my bravado-based mindset automatically connected outwardly through my senses to the mindsets in the collective society. The purpose of the collective mindset was to control and ensure the automatic want in my mind should continue to nurture my reflected bravado mind. My thoughts aligned perfectly with the external collective thoughts of society.

I broke down these different patterns of collective thinking into the hierarchal based thinking accepted by society as the powerful correct thinking based on the right and the wrong of society:

The collective conscious acceptance of power and the powerful.

The collective conscious thinking of whom and what is weak.

The collective conscious thinking of what is healthy and unhealthy.

The collective conscious thinking of who is superior and who is inferior.

The collective conscious thinking of what or who is conformed to society and distinguish the non-confirmed as unacceptable.

The collective conscious acceptance of the supreme power of education.

The collective conscious acceptance of the inferiority of the un-educated thinking.

The collective conscious acceptance of the automatic difference between people.

The collective conscious acceptance of the white race is superior, and the black race is less.

The collective conscious acceptance of the brown race is inferior.

The collective conscious acceptance of the yellow race was less again.

The collective conscious acceptance of the red race was less again.

The collective conscious acceptance of a superior, dominant religious mindset.

As I re-fitted all of this newly acquired knowledge into the particular aspects of my mind, I began to find glimmers of insight into how my mind worked. I started to understand the rotation and spins of my mind perspective into the memories of learning, knowledge and power, which was away from the sensory awareness of my heart chakra I was seeking within me. I finally began to find clarity and reason for my depression as the shadows, and their darkness began their reveal for healing.

I saw I had automatically built my mind to imitate how my perceptions recognised or interpreted the powerful collective mindset. When I flipped my perspective inwards to observe my inner mind, I saw that my perceived thinking of 'weak' people allowed me to reject or dismiss them automatically. These automatic, dismissive actions and reactions in my mind also dismissed or rejected the weakness in my mind. My perceptions of 'strong' people's thoughts became my thoughts in my mind. I absorbed the imprints of their strengths automatically, and I now recognised that in taking on their perceived strengths, I had also inherited their invisible emotions, their spiritual imprints, and made them mine. I saw my automatic projections and perceptions formed an open pathway to similar energies of the collective consciousness related directly to my child-mind learning and functioning.

The efficiency of how my perceptive skills created and fuelled my mental barriers within my mind is a staggering insight to my new enlightened perceptions.

Light permitted me to observe my child mind as I grew up. I saw how I automatically accepted the implanted ideas, suggestions, and thoughts every day by automatically accepting the opinions and thinking from adults and my peers. These adults, particularly my parents, my teachers, parish priests, and my family, subjected the child-me to belittling and threatening behaviour. As a child, I did not question these people, their opinions or their behaviour. I accepted in my mind what they said was 'right.' They were 'right' in that their voices were powerful. I can see that I cared about all these people automatically in my child mind. I assumed they cared about me. The child-me accepted their opinions of me and society automatically, and the child-me accepted that my feelings were wrong.

I saw my automatic habit of repeating a viewpoint or an idea I believed was reliable or knowledgeable and therefore acceptable to a conversation. I saw I re-voiced it automatically without questioning its integrity. In doing so, I rejected the core of me, my truth.

I saw I had automatically begun to build a childlike, silent, angry resentment within my mind that festered in my relationships and how I felt towards society. This angry resentment in my mind shaped me to become what these people told me I should be in their opinions. My automatic angry resentment built my inner mind into a reality of self-abuse. My mind seemed riddled with pain and insecurity that I automatically masked by my bravado perspective. I seemed frozen in an assumed passivity that lulled me into believing my ignorance was my life.

I can see how I became abrasive and acted out my bravado from my negative learning to please society, particularly my father. The child-me desperately wanted to feel loved, be accepted, be recognised, feel wanted, be approved of, and be included by other people. How or when did the bright, sparkling child identify herself as a densely pained child of twisted thinking? I don't have any memories of living as a sparkling happy child. I saw this dense pained, twisted child-thinking that did not permit me to study or mature in my thoughts manifest in my awareness. I saw her resistance emblazoned into my mind that blocked her from accepting any adult direction. I can now see that the child me felt afflicted by society, and the adult me reacted in the way I thought society had hurt me. The child me and young adult me projected my automatic resentment in my angry responses, angry outbursts, angry reactions, dismissive curses, and name-calling outwards towards adults and the community in general. I blamed people for my inadequacies and then competed with people in childish ways to succeed and be better than them. When my mother died, her sister – my aunt – told me that she thought the river would carry us all. I understood back then that she was speaking in metaphorical terms.

Thirty years later, I recognised I had instantly and automatically developed a crazy thought of protection in my mind to ensure that the river would not carry us. I can now see I had engaged a tremendous, almost irrational automatic resistance in my mind to my aunt's prophecy. I had automatically built a massive protective shield in my mind around my siblings. I recognised my protective shield in my bravado mind when I saw I was automatically worrying about all of them even though they never asked me to worry about them. This automatic shield denied them their unique responsibilities and their need to accept and take full responsibility for their lives, their feelings, thoughts, emotions, actions, and behaviour in my mind. I was automatically saving them from the flood of my aunt's river.

Light awareness enhanced my ability to detach from this automatic barrier, and I began to stop worrying and fretting automatically about my siblings. I have been able to cut them loose from my mind and let them be adults living by their own choices. I don't need to take responsibility for them and prove that we are not the weak people she perceived us to be.

"God, who am I?" I asked.

What a mess I am.

I tried to maintain a Light perspective within me amidst the revelations of all this pain, anxiety and emotional turbulence. I began to accept that my healing journey required me to travel into the darkness of my mind and emotions. I also saw my automatic instant ability to default to my childhood thinking was causing me considerable difficulty. I did not understand why I lost my Light perspective so quickly. These massive, learned barriers that alienated me from my unique self and life in general, did not belong in my heart's intentions that reflected my new Light awareness.

I began to accept my awareness was inspiring me to detach from society's collective consciousness and the thought patterns I had adapted in my mental barriers. I needed to detach from my child-like bravado mind.

I needed to build boundaries that aligned with the purpose of my Light awareness. I accepted I needed to take full responsibility for myself, my awareness, my intuitiveness, my feelings, my knowledge, and how I used my words. I needed to ensure that I used words and language correctly to portray my healing message and reflect my Light intention and purpose. I also needed to alter my thoughts, actions, reactions, and whole behaviour to reflect this Light awareness.

I started anew from my Light perspective in educating and restructuring my mind into a new dynamic with a higher intention and a higher original purpose. I began using my higher perspective of Light to detach from my bravado mind and the collective consciousness. Very quickly, I became conscious of how effective my boundaries of Light worked both physically and mentally.

I was stunned to discover that my Light boundary application worked amazingly well in separating my bravado mind from the collective conscious thinking and my bravado thinking from my Light awareness. I also became aware of how people's anger worked within me.

I consciously put a Light boundary of detachment between my heart consciousness and the angry person. This simple process of disciplined detachment highlighted to me how other people's anger controlled me in my mind. Their anger was a forceful, controlling mental weapon they indiscriminately and automatically projected towards me that triggered my fear of them in my mind. My fear of them activated my internal anger, which automatically connected to their external anger. I was stunned when I saw that I had created a similar weapon of unknown anger in my mind that enabled me to control people.

How deep was my anger? Which anger should I begin to heal? The revelation of this invisible anger frustrated me, frustrated my control, and frustrated my healing process. The Light showed it to be a massive mental block. As I became conscious of how angry I felt within myself, I placed a boundary of Light between my Light awareness and my learned child-mind and bravado anger. This process stopped the automated free flow of negative, angry emotions from the external collective mindset into my mind. I discovered that this free flow of negativity between minds helped support and contain me in my anger.

I began to see the other blocks of my mental barriers that were stalling the development of my healing process. For example, when I thought I had applied my Light boundary to an angry thought pattern I was endeavouring to release and heal, I felt frustrated and confused as the healing was not happening. I did not realise my Light perspective that I required to heal and release had dropped in vibration and had regressed to the fear of my learning. I did not recognise it or know it. I had to eventually retrace my thinking over and over until I recognised that my action of intention had become an automatic action. I revealed I had *assumed* that I had applied my Light boundary to this thought pattern. I had *assumed* I was healing.

I finally acknowledged that I was not detaching from a thought pattern, and I was not separating it from my bravado mind. I saw I was trying to build a Light awareness on top of my learned automatic assumed thought patterns, which does not work. The practice of inner self-discipline in my awareness was a complex process.

I began to see the assumed block of my bravado mind's attitude that I was a disciplined, independent, solid, and reliable person. This thinking was an entitled mindset I had created in the shadow of the collective consciousness, which haunted my efforts to work in the healing vibrations in my new Light awareness.

This insight helped me understand that I needed to reveal and unravel deeper thought patterns that I was unaware existed in my mind. I intuited that I needed to identify the depth of the invisible emotions contained in my mental barriers. I needed to recognise emotions of familiarity, of comfort that I was automatically seeking and regressing to in my mind. I reverted to my memory of when my father banished me from home, my family, and my mother to find this depth. I began to reflect on my journey and my behaviour when I arrived in the city.

I saw how I had regressed deeper in my new adult bravado thinking. I can see my mother's passive influences became more potent within me as I learned to live silently, internally in my thoughts as I tried to self-start my life as an adult. I kept what I thought to myself. I knuckled down, found a job and joined my older sister and her flatmates in their flat.

Now I can see I automatically relied on my sister and her friends for companionship. I was alone and lonely. I was distrustful of people, particularly men. I found it hard to fit into the city.

My relationship with my father ended so cruelly and suddenly, it cured me of any notion in my mind that I may have been a strong person or even a person of any worth.

My automatic survival instincts grew stronger as I replaced my father's control and dominance with my employer's power and dominance. This dynamic required similar behaviours of compliance, obedience, and duty from me. My employer's energies were similar to my father's energies. I recognised this at the time. It added to my frustrations and feelings of being stuck. I was meeting different people, different faces, and different voices, yet with similar mindsets to my father. Naturally, my emotions towards my father manifested in my automatic responses. I struggled to fit into the workforce. My sense of collective mental responsibility, along with an immature and overburdened work ethic, frustrated me into and out of dead-end jobs. I had this great impatience and intolerance towards management when they seemingly demanded less of me than I wanted to give. My mantra way back then to myself was, "Why can't they see the right way to do a thing?" My right way was my father's way. I did not understand then that there are many ways of working. Many years into my working career, I discovered more detached and relaxed work ethics and more efficient working methods than the work ethic I had inherited.

Naturally, in my bravado mind, I analysed my bosses as this or that. I justified my thoughts and my thinking with a tirade of unsaid frustration and anger that went into a silent automatic free flow of thinking in my mind. I often walked away from my job, silently telling my employer to stick it. Around this time, I also met my husband. I fell in love and married him. In this relationship, I felt loved. I felt safe. I felt content and secure for a long time. Naturally, as day follows night, my marriage revealed its hiding places, and they became too uncomfortable for me to bear. The shadows of me began to appear in my automatic behaviour.

These reflections were mainly of negative, influenced bravado responses and behaviour. I was alerted in my meditations to the spiralling out of control behaviour I was engaging in my bravado mind. The downward spiral into those parts of my mind was crippling me emotionally and mentally. I thought I had or I assumed I had discarded or rejected my unwanted feelings and weaknesses, that I was rid of them. I was once again shocked to realise and understand the journey of my regression. I became conscious of my insecurity by identifying my desperate neediness for complete security. I was fuelling my internal paralysis by drinking. My inebriated state of mind allowed me to think of reckless notions as I dared to test myself or other people from my double passive mind perspective. This behaviour was destructive and harmful. After my divorce, my loneliness drove me to continue with my reckless conduct.

Eventually, from a new awareness of Light, I understood that I had to heal my want for security. I needed to become a whole person in Light consciousness without experiencing or facilitating sexual, emotional, or spiritual pain. I was a social drinker, nevertheless, I recognised that it had fed into my passivity when I stopped drinking. I saw I was passive, not just emotionally, but I was passive mentally, sexually, and spiritually. I was passive in most of my behaviour. Passivity shrouded me in almost every aspect of my life. Passivity secured and protected me and validated me in the absence of self-esteem and self-confidence. Passivity helped me remain the same as other people and permitted me to be part of the crowd. Passivity allowed me to continue my drinking and carefree, happy evenings without understanding the implicated damage to my Light awareness and my responsibility towards my heart chakra and my higher self.

I recognised my childlike reactions of crying, especially if someone asked me to express my opinion or if I had to speak about how I felt. This lack of expression revealed itself in my healing career. I had no confidence in my intuitive answers to questions from people, and for a while, I was happy to ask them to pose these questions to our mentor. When they returned to our group with answers from him, I still did not give my opinion. Instead, I would say, "Did he say that?" or "I don't believe you – did he say that?"

I also recognised my automatic passivity in my false humility. "Did I say that? I don't remember?" or "Did I do that?" I recognised my timid behaviour. If I heard a noise at night, I would lay in bed in terror, waiting for the next step, the next sound. If I saw a spirit, particularly during the night, I would curse and swear at them to go away. I recognised this same passivity in my fear pattern when I had to challenge my children's teachers. Particularly at the annual parent/teacher meetings when the teachers would talk to me from behind a desk about my children's abilities and behaviour. I would silently listen from my seat opposite them, but I was reacting in my passive defensive anger in my inner mind, and I rarely ever questioned them.

Instead, in my thoughts, I was arguing silently with them, asking them massive questions. For example, "Why can't you do your job and teach my children the how and the why? Why can't you break down and explain the maths theory or the verbs or teach the science in a clear and understandable language for the children to absorb and learn? Why do you expect my children to learn off books of theories while you fail them by not explaining theories so that they can understand those theories?" I can now see I should have challenged these teachers or the education system. Nevertheless, I can also see how I automatically regressed to the forgotten frustrated pain I experienced in my childhood and the experiences of humiliation and shame my teachers imprinted in my mind. I didn't know that I was my automatic self then, pleasing and not upsetting the hierarchy.

I recognised a deeper level of my automatic passivity when Light revealed a considerable barrier of a hidden fear of potential losses in my bravado mind. I needed to break down the potential losses into the single potential losses or fears accumulated together in this dense barrier in my mind. As I reflected on this barrier, I began to see that for all of my married life, I feared the loss of my husband through early death, the loss of his health. I feared the loss of my own life and the loss of my children's lives. I feared the potential loss of our business, home, money, and the potential fear of failing. I can now see that these fears had little prospect of manifesting in my life because my husband and I both worked so hard to survive. Where and how were these losses created, and what influenced them?

Nevertheless, they were real fears that influenced my mind, unknowingly and invisibly.

As a young wife and mother, I recognised that I was terrified that my husband would abandon his family and leave me alone to fend for us. I feared for how we would survive. I realised I had developed an intuitive over-protective coping skill in my mind that fuelled this barrier. I recognised my automatic behaviour revealed an over-anxiousness, an over-indulged type of mother and wife. I thought I was giving the impression of easy-going in my bravado mind, but I was the opposite. I saw my behaviour was powerfully controlling of them.

I was influencing them with what I had assumed to be rational logic before discovering my irresponsible, entitled expectations of control. This unknown control defined my rule, my love, my sacrifice, my purpose, my hopes, my intention, my way for them.

In return, my bravado thinking entitled me to expect their compliance, their duty, their loyalty, their love from them.

Light also revealed the complicated relationship with money in my mind. I saw I irrationally feared money. For example, I feared not having any money for food. I did not take responsibility for money. I wasn't conscious of this fear in my thoughts. During my divorce, I understood that I had abdicated my responsibilities for handling money to my husband during our marriage.

As I released fear, I revealed further fears. For example, I was frightened of power. I was afraid of dying. I revealed an irrational fear of starvation. I revealed the fear of isolation and rejection of me by other people. I revealed I was terrified of God, of hell and the devil. I revealed a fear of poverty, loneliness and anger. I was fearful of not being loved. I feared my sexuality.

Overall, I saw that I endeavoured to control my anger in my bravado mind. I tried to cleanse it from my thoughts and feelings, to reassure myself that I was not an angry or cross person. I knew I was afraid of other people's judgment, and I did not want to be seen or remembered as an angry person. I wanted people to believe I was a strong positive person. I was also conscious I did not want my children to remember me as angry, in the same way I remembered my father's anger. I can see that this automatic containment of my thinking and emotions kept my mind in an energised pressure cooker-style confinement, ready to explode at any moment.

The trigger that unleashed my unknown suppressed anger came from my husband's affidavit during our divorce process. After reading it, I remember I physically collapsed as I felt my stomach cave in, and I lost power in my legs. I was in complete disbelief and shock as my body shook and my mind imploded. I felt empty.

If his affidavit truthfully reflected how he felt in the marriage, then my intuition about our marriage was accurate. It confirmed that I had lived in a hopeless void within marriage. I recognised we were both failures, not just me. For several weeks, I felt I could not speak as my voice felt choked. "You cannot treat me like this!" I often raged at him. My anger fuelled my mind, and I became paranoid about my husband's behaviour. Suddenly one morning, I woke up understanding that I was playing his game and his solicitor's game. I knew I would lose their game. I realised that the only way I could help myself was to detach from him, his friends, and his solicitor.

As my senses calmed, I realised I had to fight this divorce parody through the courts. I needed to trust the judicial system.

I detached from my husband and my divorce. I stopped fighting with him in my mind. I felt inspired by Light to disentangle the powerful negative emotions we were fighting and blaming each other with that fuelled our pain and blame.

I needed to accept full responsibility for the emotions that were in my mind. I needed to accept that the anger I raged in was indeed my anger and frustration. I had entrusted my life to him under the hand of God in my marriage vows, however, with the insight of my divorce affidavit, I felt I had wasted my life.

I began to see that it was in my failure to voice my feelings that I betrayed the core of my essence that permitted him to betray me. On reflection, I saw my devotion to him, how I became dependant on him, how I had trusted him, the way I believed in him became a reliance on him. I also relied on him for my identity, my role, my security, and my purpose. When he pulled the plug on my status, I was nothing. I witnessed my strength seep away. I was a shell of a human being. I also felt challenged, if not ashamed, by the depth and severity of my pain. I can say in truth that these revelations were harrowing for me to bear and to accept because I resisted them as my weakness, my failure, my vulnerability. My Light awareness finally began to understand the severity and the depth of my chronic pain. I prayed for the courage to begin the process of releasing and transmuting all the powerlessness. As I began to identify my powerlessness within me, I began to find deep hurt and pain. For the first time, I recognised and validated my suppressed feelings of darkness, betrayal, rejection, fear and loss.

I reverted to my childhood to begin to disentangle my family memories and reveal my suppressed feelings. I particularly sought out the memories of sibling arguments, the fights and the painful episodes that impacted me mentally and emotionally.

I remembered when two of my sisters told me that they feared conversations with me as they felt that they had to walk on eggshells when in my company. Neither one could say this from an individual perspective – they needed to cluster together to attack.

"Listen, and accept what they say," I heard in my inner mind. I had observed my bravado intention was to present myself to the world as a well-rounded, open, accepting, achieving person. My bravado intention was not an honest or accurate perception of me. My sisters had felt challenged by my anger. I began the detachment process from my sisters and our conversation.

I began my self-healing by not responding to them automatically and taking a step away from my automatic responses. During our discussion, my Light awareness intuited me to not argue with my sisters. I carefully chose my answer to them to reflect my Light perspective.

It was a long couple of years before my mental resistance and defensiveness allowed this argument's real emotions to emerge. On this occasion, I recognised that my frustrations were a major block in my mind. My frustrations blocked me from seeing or recognising my anger. I intuited that my anger was not a single blanket of angry emotions. It was made up of many different angry emotions that in themselves contained different vibrations of pain. Before I could recognise my anger to heal it, I needed to release my frustrations consciously. I saw that my frustrations formed a dense mist within my mind, clouding my thinking and feeling.

I tried many ways to release my frustrations. For example, I walked them out, I tried running and cycling. Eventually, I intuited that my frustrations had to release through my throat chakra. As I meditated, I asked Light how I was going to do that. I saw a glimpse of me roaring in meditation that helped me develop a therapy that began releasing pressurised frustrations from within my mind.

I started by opening my mouth in a safe environment, like an empty park and trying to roar. I could not do it. I could only whimper, which reflected my lack of voice.

I focused on finding inspiration that would help me to expand the unblocking of my frustrations in my meditations. During several meditations, I began to put together a configuration of chakras that felt safe to me. I consciously engaged this alignment of chakras before I tried to roar out my frustrations again. My chakras' alignment provided a safety structure for me to begin to release my known and unknown frustrations without flooding my mind in my unknown amassed emotional pain.

I developed my therapy as follows: I connected my intention to release frustrations into the Light in my heart chakra. I focused the Light downwards from my heart chakra through my internal chakra system. I connected it to my feet chakras. I then exited the Light through my feet chakras to enter the earth energies to ground me. I reconnected to the Light in my heart, and this time, I raised it upwards through my upper chakras. I exited the Light from my crown chakra and raised it upwards to find the highest vibration of Light to support me. I asked the highest Light vibration for help and support to inspire me to let go of frustrations, release and heal my emotions. Only then did I proceed with the healing.

I stood my feet very firmly on the ground with my knees bent. I placed my hands on my hips. I bent my upper body and tilted my head downwards to look into my solar plexus chakra. I inhaled a deep breath of air through my nose, and as I did, I imagined I was also inhaling Light. I held the breath and the Light in my lungs for a count of five. While I was counting, I intentionally straightened my body. I threw back my head, I began to exhale my breath slowly through my open mouth and then I roared using the power of the exhale to release my frustrations.

I needed to repeat the routine many times before I sensed the process of release beginning for me. When I finished roaring, I grounded my chakras in Light. Afterwards, I always feel washed out and exhausted. I believe this is normal after such an exercise.

After I began to vent my frustrations, I found clarity in my thoughts that helped me reveal the different core emotions I needed to engage during my healing sessions. I needed to allow myself to feel my emotions by experiencing them through my Light boundaries. I needed to accept my emotions, and I needed to take personal responsibility for them before I could begin to transmute or release them.

Plenty of rest and sleep are essential requirements to my healing process.

The following critical reflection came between my daughter and me – there were two. The first one happened when we were both sitting in church during Mass. My daughter was about eight years old.

A young girl of similar age to my daughter was standing on the altar of our church doing a reading. In the middle of the reading, her face froze into an image of her anxiety. I reached for my daughter's hand, and she whispered to me, "Mum, I feel like that sometimes." My heart instantly sank to my toes. Oh God, what can I do to help her? I felt so helpless at that moment. I felt such a failure as a mother and as a person. How did this happen to my precious little girl? What had I said to her, which of my actions had resulted in her feeling this turmoil and anxiety? I had thought that this type of anxiety belonged to other people and not to us.

While we were cooking dinner that afternoon, I revisited the conversation of what happened to the girl on the altar.

I explained how I thought the young girl was nervous about reading in front of all the people. The nervous feelings grew as she read. I explained that I thought the nervous feelings became too big in her mind, she lost her focus, and panicked in her mind. It was her nervous feelings that thwarted her intention to read and speak.

I explained to my daughter that I felt the young girl had not been coached sufficiently in her coping skills to survive the stress of the considerable task her teacher had asked of her. After all, grown men and women suffer from nervous feelings, although they draw on life experiences and their boundaries to cope with them.

I asked my daughter if she remembered when her nervous feelings started. Did she know what set them off? Did she remember the last time she felt her nervous feelings? I asked her if she could tell me when the worst feelings happened for her. She could not find answers to my questions, so I changed the subject from her nervous feelings, and I began to show her all the positive stuff that she could identify within herself. I listed out everything she enjoyed doing and all the tasks she quickly completed and enjoyed. For example, she loved to cook, dance, play tennis, music, and swim. She loved to curl up and read. She was a great helper in the office and our home. She was a great friend, a great sister, a great cousin, and above all, she was a terrific daughter loved and cherished by both of her parents.

I knew I needed to keep her perspective separate from her school experiences and her friend's experiences on the altar. I also explained to her that nervous feelings could grow into anxiety. I said I believed it was just a blip in thinking that needed tweaking. We promised each other that we would try and fix it. Therefore, we agreed to work to recognise events or thoughts that were causing it. At that time, I was not confident in my intuition as I had only begun to scratch the surface of my anxieties and healing.

My daughter and I decided to have chats about her feelings of fears when they happened. I checked her diet for allergies to ensure that her food was not a contributing factor to her mental tension. We realised from lots of chats and discussions that she felt fear sometimes filling her mind. It became apparent to me that sometimes it was my thoughts that were affecting her. I began to observe my behaviour to find the factors I projected from my mind to contribute to her anxieties.

Many years later, my daughter worked in teams of people and was required to speak to them to present her ideas and how they worked. During this time, she became aware of her anxieties again. When she talked to me about her concerns, I trusted my intuition. I knew I could help her, and she trusted me to help her.

The anxiety manifests in her mind as a sense of loss that makes her think she will forget her words. This loss in her communication or her inability to express herself only becomes visible to her colleagues as her face reddens in embarrassment at her perceived fear of failure. Continued efforts to communicate with clarity and confidence, to express how she truly feels will help her detach from her anxiety and heal its root eventually.

In my efforts to help my daughter to build her confidence, I became aware I was also self-healing the damaged daughter aspects within my mind. Her anxieties reflected the inner mental anxieties in my mind that were previously unknown to me, yet they significantly contributed to the way I communicated at that time. During this period, I had started to facilitate meditations and workshops. I needed to find my voice, confidence, and self-esteem that would permit me to speak my truth, my Light. Instead, I found that my voice was crippled, choked by emotion that blocked me in my efforts to find my truth. Speaking my truth is an ongoing process for me. I find it challenging in my awareness, especially if I am talking about the pain of my healing journey.

The second insight that impacted me occurred during my second spiritual reading with my mentor. After lengthy deliberations within my thoughts, it transpired that this reading was more about the father aspects of my mind than my relationship with my father. I did not know this at the time of the reading.

My mentor said to me, "Your father asks why you are putting your daughter on the stage when she is not ready to be there?"

I said defensively, "I think you have got this wrong because my daughter is not into drama at all. What's more, she is not in the least dramatic and not interested in the stage."

He just smiled at me and did not engage my opinion, and he repeated the sentence very calmly. I sucked in my defensive thoughts. I started to think that this was rubbish and not at all as good as the first reading I'd had with him. It was months later when it suddenly clicked in my thoughts that I was pushing my daughter to grow up, to be out there in the world at too young an age. This clarity occurred after a tense conversation she and I had about her education. She found it challenging to memorise her subjects.

It was unfortunate that our education system demanded that children learn off and remember reams of texts and repeat their remembered learning during exams. It meant that they did not necessarily have to learn the breakdown of their subjects' theories or understand them creatively or otherwise. To retain learning in her mind, she had to repeatedly read text for hours to recall it for exams.

I knew my daughter was exceptionally bright, and she was alert and curious. When I sat down with her and explained chores, she understood instantly. For example, she often helped me out in my office. I showed her how to do the different tasks I required. She grasped them immediately. She was proficient at office work from a young age and had no difficulty applying herself to it. She often sat in the reception area and handled the office's procedure as if she were a person ten years older.

When she was younger, about nine or ten years old, she took an interest in cooking. It seemed to come naturally to her. She would lay out everything she needed on the kitchen table. She baked in front of us and told us, her audience, what she was doing and why she was doing it. I felt she was so confident in her personality. I asked my husband if he would finance a video of her baking. I believed we could sell it to TV companies. She was such a natural girl – she was keen, funny, and very efficient in her baking. I felt sure that the video was a dead cert for success.

Thirty years ago, there were no children's cooking shows, but now they are trendy. I knew and trusted that she had tremendous abilities and capabilities. When it came to her studying, I felt that something was wrong. I was unable to help her. I could not set up a study practice and show her the different ways to study because I had never studied in my school years. I felt frustrated and angry at the difficulties that were building for her.

I began to get impatient with the routine she had engaged in that ensured she passed her Junior Certificate exams with honours. I felt that she was pushing herself too far, involving a work ethic that was too severe for her. I suggested that she think about leaving school and developing a career in business, as she was outstanding when she worked in our company. She cried bitterly at my suggestion.

She looked at me through her tears and said, "Mum, I am trying hard here! Why can't you believe me?"

Instantly, I saw my limitations reflected in my responses to her, showing me that I had made no effort in my education. I was intolerant of her ambition, in her need to learn at whatever cost to her. I was not supporting her in her study. I was telling her what to do, what I thought was best for her.

I recognised that I was encouraging her to opt out of education as I had opted out. Was I unconsciously pushing my daughter out into the world as my father had pushed me out? Was I keeping my daughter at my level of education and within my mental limitations? Did I want to deny her the chance to be different to me? I was applying the harsh, severe judgement that my father had passed on me when I was a young girl. Was I passing this judgement on her? Was I mothering my child as my father had parented me?

Ouch.

I sensed pain. We hugged until we calmed down and stopped crying. I promised to support her in every way to help her make her study easier. She went on to college and achieved a master's degree in her favourite subjects seven years later.

This reflection revealed my banks of frustration and disappointment with my teachers that had built up into an invisible, negative undercurrent of frustrated energies, influencing disrespect for education and teachers automatically in my mind. I recognised the frustrated and disrespectful thought patterns regarding my automatic rejections of the academic world in our society. They appear not challenged by anyone or anything. They are supremely confident of what they think they know. I recognised I carried a deep automatic hatred for school and teachers.

I realised the limitations in my learning that my smiling face masked. I projected 'happy' to hide my inadequacies and my pain. My mask was a combination of humour and anger. Through my efforts in writing this book, I am finally transmuting a lot of my learned thinking. When I started writing, I was unaware of the difference between the mind and the heart within myself. I was ignorant that I had a multi-dimensional mindset and a Light aspect of a very high vibration. This particular reading from my mentor reflected my mind. It revealed a massive ignorance in my mind. It also showed my ignorant thoughts and behaviour towards my daughter that was causing her to hurt. The healing and transmutation of this revelation in my mind became an invaluable step to my healing. I changed my mental perspective on her education. I began to support and treat her as an adult. I stopped automatically pushing her as had been my habit in the past.

I remember another insightful, life-changing incident I had in the centre where I worked. My mentor is a highly acknowledged, famous, respected spiritual healer and tutor. He is a published writer, a spiritual healing tutor, an accomplished spiritual healer and an accurate and respected clairvoyant. As I said earlier, he was the person that gave me support and direction in my efforts to change and heal myself. I assumed I was accepting and respectful of him when I worked with him in his centre.

What happened in my mind for the first three or so years of my spiritual healing career? I stepped into his centre to change me and to become a spiritual healer of the highest integrity. Instead, I unwittingly adopted the same unknown automatic supportive role of who I was as a wife, a mother, a sister and a daughter. I engaged my healing awareness and insight automatically when I put myself in the shadow of his success.

I recognised that I automatically thought I was a lesser person than him in every way. When I revealed my thinking and fears about him, I felt stupid, disappointed, and vulnerable in myself.

I had automatically perceived him and his work from my immature supporter role. It took several painful lessons for me to begin to understand my supporter role, my pain, and my hidden learned shadows. I revealed the reason I regressed so profoundly into the depths of my child-mind at such a critical junction in my life, and especially when I so consciously wanted to change. I began to see I had negatively interpreted every instance when my mentor did not ask me to support him in the automatic manner that I had learned how to support men in particular. When I realised he was independent of me in every way, I felt massively challenged by him. In my bravado mind, I realised I needed to feel his dependence, reliance, and need for me so I could feel I was of value to him or myself. This relationship left me feeling inadequate, even unwanted. I felt alone. I felt isolated as I struggled in my spiritual healing and facilitating careers. I felt my inferiority and isolation again when he told me that my lack of education was a block to my spiritual healing career progression. In other words, I was unacceptable to him and to the NFSH (National Federation of Spiritual Healers of Great Britain) healing body to train as a tutor. This perceived lack of support and total rejection of me, the healer, drove me deeper into the hurt and the shadows in my mind. I could have blamed others and felt justified in pointing fingers, but I knew I had painful aspects of myself to recognise, unfold, heal, and release. I had my intention to work in Light, which was unaffected by the dominant and controlling judgements of society's hierarchy.

A few years later, I can see I was so lucky and protected by the universe that day when he said I was not tutor material. I can see I fitted perfectly into the supportive role of helping others in the centre.

From my supportive perspective, I would not have discovered that this was a learned role in my mind and not me. I was very comfortable and very content supporting and introducing people to their spiritual journeys. I can see I felt empowered with what I felt from witnessing their spiritual awakenings. I now believe that my mentor was courageous that day in saying no to my request to learn to be a tutor.

The universe has inspired my journey since then. It has directed me to seek and nurture my higher self. I was very much ignorant of the existence of my higher self, which I currently call my Light awareness. I had automatically thought I was reaching higher levels within myself by learning to become a tutor. The very painful rejection by my mentor drove me to ask more questions about myself and my mind. My realisation that glass ceilings of limitations exist even on my spiritual journey was inspiring for me. My automatic persistence of living in my ignorant shadow-supporter identity drove me from the centre and the people I loved.

I intentionally exposed my vulnerabilities without protection, conscious that their exposure within my awareness would force me to look at whatever shape these shadows and weaknesses took.

As my healing progressed, the continuing transmutation of mental pain to Light began to lift my mind vibration. I became aware of very subtle changes within me. I felt confidence expand within my Light awareness. It led me to trust and believe in myself, and that developed my self-esteem. The emergence of Light from my heart chakra influenced my confidence and self-esteem that permitted me to lift and change the vibration of my mind.

During my meditations, my higher Light perspective revealed the invisible spirit identities that had lodged in the lower vibrations of my mind. They had found their hiding places in the comfort and familiarity of the lower aspects of my mind that provided them with the protection and security they needed to continue to exist in their spirit world. These spirits came from the different existences of their physical journeys. Some of their lives went back to prehistoric times.

The healing and the release from these spirits' imprint and influences helped me understand their blanket influences were negative barriers in my mind. Their presence had blighted my efforts to be positive and to heal myself. I recognised their persistent repetitive thoughts of needing desperately to survive masked their overwhelming fearful emotions that fuelled similar emotional, painful vibrations in my mind.

For example, I remember one spirit manifesting in a meditation of an impoverished woman trying to patch a roof on a cold, wet, wintry afternoon. She seemed to be the strong one and yet was not strong at all. I sensed her pain and anxiety about her children as they lay inside her house, dying of starvation. When I saw her children, they were dead.

I can recognise that her driving need to survive and protect her children was similar to my driving need to

survive in my life and protect my children. I also understood her survival drive masked her emotions of dread
and fear at losing her children. Her fearful emotions impacted my mind and my emotions of similar vibrations.

Another meditation revealed a house on fire and an
impoverished woman, once again on her own, trying to
protect her children and keep them alive. They huddled in
the mud with only a blanket to protect them from the cold
and wet weather. She seemed unaware that her children
were dead. Her passivity shrouded her overwhelming
fears for their survival, but also her denial of and fear of
death. Her passivity and her fears impacted my fears and
emotions of similar vibrations in my mind.

Another meditation revealed a spirit woman tied by
ropes in a wooden cage. It was hard to separate her from
the initial thought I had that she was a wild dog. With
careful questioning from the group facilitator, I eventually found a woman caked in mud. I identified her suffering, her isolation, her rejection, her fear, and her rage. She
was fighting to survive imprisonment by her tribe. She
felt abandoned, isolated, and unloved.

I clearly remember when I felt unwell on another afternoon of our meditation evening. I was feeling very intense pain in my chest. Nevertheless, I decided to head
into the centre.

I had just sat on my chair in the group circle, and I
closed my eyes to connect to Light. Instantly, I began to
shiver with the cold. I physically could not control the

cold that was gripping the whole of me. The meditation began, and Linda, our facilitator, asked me if I was ok.

"No, I feel I am freezing," I said. The instant I acknowledged the cold, I felt my feet heavy and cold. I looked down at them, and they were in layers of what looked like cloth sacking tied with a cord. It seemed I was walking in the snow. I looked outwards at the endless snow. I turned to look back – all I could see was snow. I was entirely on my own. There was a spirit man in severe pain manifesting in my awareness. Linda asked who he was, and he answered he was an Arctic explorer looking for the North Pole. As the man spoke through me, I felt his pain in my chest pain gain momentum. He said, "I am in pain. It's like a hot knife burning through my chest."

Linda spoke to him and helped him to release his pain. Eventually, his image transmuted to Light, and he moved into the care of his Light guide. As he did, the pain in my chest eased and finally cleared.

The driving perspective in the explorer's memory pushed his mind on a continued spirit walk for centuries before he was ready to ask for help to move on to another spiritual dimension.

In the same way I had felt the cold, I felt incredible heat and a sense of burning one evening in meditation. I smelled smoke. I was becoming uncomfortable in my meditative state. Linda, the facilitator, asked me if I was ok.

"No, I am on fire," I said. As soon as I acknowledged the burning, I was looking through a spirit woman's eyes.

216

I saw her body tied to a stake and was about to be burned. The fire was beginning to catch my feet. There were people around the fire shouting and roaring. Linda quickly sensed the fear and began to speak with the spirit woman. She asked her why she was being burned alive. The spirit said it was because she was a healer. During this revelation, I needed to be determined and focused on my detachment from the spirit. Eventually, the spirit transmuted and went with her Light guides. I released the imprint of her colossal panic and the fear of her impending brutal, vicious death that could so quickly have become fear, terror and pain in my mind.

I understood these spirit existences had wrapped around my mental energies, drawing their comfort and familiarity from the vibrations of my mind. I was horrified when I realised that the spirits were also fuelling my perspective in fear and irrational thoughts. I saw that these external spirits had hugely influenced me and contained my thinking in the lower vibrations of pain and thoughts. I was not aware of or conscious of these static and negative influences existing in and fuelling my mind.

Light intuited me to accept responsibility for all of my mind and its vibrations. I had to take responsibility for my life to date, knowing that I had been living like a robot in my bravado mind. My thoughts and emotions were driven unknowingly by invisible existences of dark, paralysing, irrational, static and toxic spiritual realities. However, these spiritual insights have enlightened and empowered my awareness of how I became and remained a victim for most of my life.

I realised I was working with the invisible, the unknown deeper dark layers of my inherited mental barriers full of memories of inherited religious and society's dogmas.

My Intuited, Interpreted Inner Mind

I reverted to my meditations and my sensed Light perspective to reveal my intuited, interpreted inner mind. I eventually accepted the series of shapes that flashed into my awareness during my meditations. I feel they adequately explained the mechanics of the family dynamic of thinking. These shapes were the symbols that helped me sense my higher self and understand my Light perspective versus the bravado mind perspective supported by collective consciousness.

The first symbols of the family dynamic came in a series of jigsaw shapes. There were ten shapes that I feel represented the ten members of my family unit during my meditations. When I fitted the pieces together to complete the jigsaw puzzle, I asked for a picture representing my family dynamic. I got an image of a forest. I pasted it on the jigsaw pieces to complete the puzzle of my family dynamic. Even though I am the seventh shape of this jigsaw or the seventh person within our family unit, my shape on the jigsaw reflected the whole forest's image. I understand that my shape of the puzzle, or me the person, contains a complete sensory picture and total memory of the original ten-piece forest jigsaw. All the other shapes or other family members have their unique sensory images with full memories of the original ten-piece forest jigsaw contained within their shapes. When all the shapes fit together, they combine to represent an image of a whole forest containing the collective mental learning of memories and emotions representing the whole family dynamic.

The powerful resources of the family dynamic automatically teach the individual members to survive, think, and feel. The family unit stands as a compelling and authoritative resource of survival that shows each child how to be physically and mentally strong. It provides a safe, secure place of learned comfort and security for each person. It compels each person to reflect the family dynamic of thinking. Each person's dynamic of thinking reveals each person's automatic thoughts and automatic behaviour that reflects how to survive, how to love, how to accept love, how to belong, how to be powerful, holy, obedient, dutiful, and loyal. Yet, each person's uniqueness within the family unit carries the Light within. Their higher self must interpret their unique sensations within the family unit as their hidden sensory, intuitive truth. The fundamental invisible difference between each person within the family unit is their unique ability to interpret their truth. Each person learns that the family unit does not require their unique truth. Each individual learns to suppress or deny their unique feelings of sensory truth and say what they have learned from the powerful family perspectives.

The family dynamic of learning is the invisible glue of thoughts and feelings that unite different people together as a whole family unit. However, the suppressed unique interpreted truth builds into banks of feelings and emotions that are fundamentally unknown to the individual mind. They manifest as the hidden pain-filled barriers within the individual's mind. When I challenged these substantial barriers within my mind, I usurped the glue that bound and balanced my family dynamic together.

I reverted to the image of my metaphoric forest to understand how my sensory reality worked. I explored the visions of the forest that came to me during my meditations. I saw the forest was a wilderness. Big trees were growing among small trees. They were overshadowing smaller trees and weaker trees. New trees were growing beside older trees. There were trees with drooping branches, trees with dead branches. Tree branches mingled with different trees. Broken branches were clinging to remain attached to their trees. There was decaying wood, decaying foliage, and protruding roots. The network of the invisible, buried roots in the earth itself all meshed and grew together underneath the earth.

The forest behaved as nature intended. The trees responded to the seasons. They bud, they blossom, and they harvest. They shed their fruit and leaves individually but at the same time, they reseed and root automatically and separately. They retreat for individual and collective protection during the winter.

I heard in my meditation that a forester must maintain a forest in continuous good health. A good forester must remove trees and offshoots of trees that have seeded too near other trees. A good forester prunes branches and removes even healthy trees for the benefit of the forest. Every tree in the forest must enjoy personal space, both above ground and underground, to grow and blossom. Each tree reflects the healthiness of the surrounding trees.

How was I going to save myself and at the same time unravel the forest within my mind? How could I create the space within my learned thinking to purge my overgrowth of trees, branches, and roots? How would I clear my space without causing further decay and further overshadowing in the surrounding forest? I focused my intention and purpose on my higher self to find answers. Finally, one evening during my meditation, I realised I was not a partial forest, even though I had taken on a whole forest's sensory knowledge.

My unique Light and sensory body manifested as the symbol of a tree during my healing and meditation. I accepted my tree was the healing tool of Light that would permit me to separate my unique senses from the forest's collective senses.

I began exploring my imaginary tree during meditation when I stepped into its trunk, and I blended my sensory body with the sensory body of the tree. From within the tree trunk, I stretched my body downwards to feel the depth and power of tree roots connected deep in the earth.

I blended my sensory feet to these roots, which helped me to stay grounded. Within the tree again, I stretched my senses upwards to feel the tree as it grew upwards. As I found the branches, I reached outwards to feel the breadth of the tree. I felt both the strength and the physical power of the energies of the tree. I also felt my senses expand into different vibrations of Light as I began to sense freedom.

It took me a while to completely trust my senses' intuition and accept that I felt the vibrations of Light that I was endeavouring to find and engage. I continued this work of trusting my sensory learning in all of my meditations. I gradually developed confidence within me that permitted me to accept that my tree provided me with the tools to create a new Light consciousness.

I finally accepted that the forest of collective trees represented my automatic intuited, learned inner mind.

I saw that it was from a small child's perspective that I automatically imitated, interpreted, and learned the deadly silence of the family dynamic. I understood it as my truth of the unsaid, and the entitled, which I automatically assumed was the truth of my family. I recognised that my senses interpreted the moods of the different silent emotions of the family dynamic. My pained imprinted face reflected the suppressed emotions within me. I repeated their opinions as my thoughts. I heard what I learned to hear. I saw what I learned to see. I began to understand the collective jumble of energies in the family forest that

I thought was my mind was not, in fact, my mind at all. I saw the inherited birthright of my family dynamic was the survival thinking of farming. Individually, we emerged from it looking physically active and capable. We were healthy, honest, and proud, programmed to work as if our very lives depended on our work.

My inner mind reality crumbled because I did not pay any attention to who I was in my mind. My mind had grown entangled and bound up with the different minds of the other members of my family unit.

During my meditations, I intuited I could clear the tangled forest energies from my mind. At about this same time, I started to interpret new awareness from the wisdom of Light.

From this perspective of enlightened awareness, I understood I needed to separate the many layers of my intuited interpreted inner mind thinking. I saw each layer was powerful support to the previous layer.

1. My Intuited unique interpretations of my Senses.
2. How I used my Senses to Interpret and Build the Thoughts in My Inner Mind.
3. My Intuited interpretations of the Power of the Family Dynamic of Thinking.
4. My Intuited Inherited Interpretation of the Family Dynamic of Thinking.
5. My Interpretation of Society's Intuitive Dynamic of Thinking.

6. My Interpretation of Society's Inherited Dynamic of Thinking.
7. My Interpreted Intuited Religious Thinking.
8. My Interpretation of my Religious Intuited Feelings.
9. My Intuited Family Dynamic of Automatic Behaviour.

1. My Intuited unique interpretations of my Senses.

I began to accept that my inner mind was created in darkness by my senses. I began to understand my inner mind darkness by recognising my unique interpretations of what I sensed as the silent and unknown interpretations I intuited from within the family dynamic. It was unknown to everyone else in the family but me. I did not know of its existence until it was revealed to my Light awareness when I began my mission to understand my inner mind.

I interpreted the influence of my intuited thinking as fear. I found this fear initially by recognising my fears within thoughts and feelings. I saw that I did not challenge people's opinions and suppressed my disagreement with their opinions. I began to understand that I did this to maintain peace within relationships.

Then I became conscious of an inner fear when I recognised my inability to assert myself, even by saying no. I needed to find the strength to say no. This no was not in disobedience or defiance. It was a no I had to say from a small place within me. It was a no I meant. It was a no that was not open for change or for pacifying. I sat and waited for the consequences of my saying no.

As I sat and waited to meet my fate, I planned how I would survive the consequences. The reaction to my no was only a shrug of the shoulders. The big question I needed to ask myself was at what stage in my early life did I learn to dismiss my feelings and opinions? What had me so frightened of authority? Why did I believe so strongly in my mind that I did not have the right to say no? What hidden, unknown fear was driving me into lower and painful parts of my mind?

I automatically accepted the thinking in my bravado mind was 'right' and was 'knowledgeable.' I saw that everything I learned that felt non-threatening to my perceptions, I automatically compartmentalised into the different segments of this mind.

For example, thoughts and feelings that automatically felt good and unchallenging to me, I knew were nice, familiar, comforting, and protective had grown to become my mind and my identity.

Secondly, I saw I automatically discarded, dismissed, or suppressed and denied unique sensations that I had learned to dislike. I learned that these sensations were weak, fearful, unacceptable, inadequate, threatening, and were surplus to the family dynamic of learning or the collective mindset.

To help me understand this flipping mechanism that twisted my senses into negative fuel for my mind, I split open a segment of my mind. I found many cells of energy. When I took away the protective and controlling membranes of learning, I found my sensory feelings of pain existed within these layers of cells. I saw all its sensations of rawness, in all its powerlessness.

I recognised how my denied sensations of unconditional love and its truth had grown unknowingly into my hurt feelings and emotions that had become my invisible powerlessness. The invisible powerlessness that I thought belonged to other people existed within me and hugely influenced my mind. My invisible powerlessness reflected my interpretation of the invisible chronic pain of my family dynamic. It was also the reflection of the pain of the collective consciousness of society.

When I released my pain, I found the truth of unconditional love that I had denied or suppressed because I didn't know it existed for me.

I also saw how my bravado perspective mechanism of 'deny and suppress' worked. For example, if I sensed a feeling of loss within me, I automatically fled its sensations to reach my learned loss instantly.

This learning will be to the comfort of familiarity that is supportive of my automatic reaction to a feeling of loss. Each time I deny, suppress, or ignore the sense of loss, I automatically create memories of loss.

After my divorce, I did not acknowledge the massive loss within me which revealed my hidden grief. My mind and body plunged into my chronic pain that manifested as physical pain. As a result, I became physically ill with different sicknesses in my body that I could not recover from, such as crippling viruses, colds, and flu. My back ached and that pain became a constant in my life. My lungs felt full, and my heart ached. My chest felt like cement.

Eventually, I surrendered to my intuition, and I accepted that I was drowning in chronic pain. I began to detach from my chronic pain by engaging my boundaries. My Light awareness showed me how the domino effect of chronic pain worked in my mind. I recognised how I created and developed my chronic pain by my automatic denial of my feelings. My denial and suppression mechanisms were the controlling and driving forces of my thinking that automatically hid my emotions in blankets of sadness, fear, loss, and trauma that completely sucked up any positivity or joy within my mind.

In essence, I can recognise now that I had no conscious knowledge of grief. I did not understand grief. Our family did not speak of grief. After my mother died, we did not speak of grief as a family of siblings. I remember someone told me not to cry during her funeral. It seems now we were all focused on my father, how we could support him and not upset him. We made plans to visit him each weekend, even though my sister lived near him and visited him most days. My brother lived and worked with him on the farm.

Nobody asked me how I was coping with the loss of my mother. I asked no one how they were dealing with the loss of their mother.

I began to heal my grief and unhappiness by accepting and recognising the heartache I felt in my whole body at the loss of my marriage and the heartache I experienced in the way my husband conducted the divorce. I became aware there were other different levels to my marriage heartache. For example, I realised the massive pain of losing my husband. He was not just my husband, he was my working partner, the security of my future, my friend, and he was the father of my children.

I felt massively injured at the easy way my husband discarded me and stopped loving me. I recognised an immense sense of failure within me because I could not reach my husband's integrity or heart. I could not find the appropriate feelings to express sufficiently and clearly to my husband how I felt, which may have reached him and inspired him to understand and respect me. I also felt I was a failure because my marriage had failed.

I became aware of other feelings of loss within me as I recognised I had lost my identity to my marriage. I had lost my sense of security. I had lost my family. I had lost my home. I realised the pain of losing my friends that disappeared out of my life favouring my husband.

When I first walked into my rented apartment, I resolved never to build a home again. I refused to buy kitchen equipment as that meant I was making a new home.

I often asked myself why I did not buy such and such, and the answer always came back to my resolution not to build a new home. This mental resolution was an automatic and substantial invisible block in my mind that I had built to protect myself from the pain at the loss of my marriage and my family home. At the time of my marriage breakup, it was a tool that helped me to survive the brutal and cruel pain, and the isolation of divorce.

At this time, I also became aware of society's hypocrisy and its subtle punishment of people like me that step outside the status quo's righteous behaviour. Society's response towards me was to isolate me. I felt its lack of support or sympathy for me in my grief.

I was lucky that I was no longer reliant on my church for spiritual support because it automatically excommunicated me. It banned me from receiving communion or partaking in their other sacraments because I broke their rules when I broke my marriage vows by seeking a divorce. This excluding action by the church became the automatic example that society copied and acted out towards me.

I compared this to how people behaved when a friend died shortly before my divorce. I saw how people reached out to the family and offered support. I also saw that most of these same people passed me, refused to talk to me or acknowledge me after my separation even though I was also suffering a considerable loss. Nobody shook my hand. Nobody sympathised with me, hugged me, or reassured me that I would be ok. I was dead to most of these people. I felt their sympathies and support lay with my husband.

When I realised that I was living my life in a haze of an unknown, intense, grieving existence, I withdrew from socialising. As a newly divorced woman, I didn't know what society expected from me. I did not know what to expect from myself. It seemed to my low self-esteem perspective that people expected me to be up for anything. For a while, I carried on my social life as I had when I was a wife.

I tried to enjoy evenings out meeting people. During these occasions, I became aware I was acutely conscious of the lack of intimacy in my life. I felt couples reflected the lack of intimacy to me. The confidence of their affection oozed intimacy to me. This reveal was so painful that I stopped socialising altogether with couples. I had accepted that I was missing the privacy of a sexual relationship, but I knew I wasn't craving sex. I also knew within my heart that sex with another person was not necessarily a precursor to finding happiness and a sense of completeness within me. I began to detach from my void of intimacy.

Through this reveal of my emotional voids, I realised I lived my life assuming. I had assumed I knew intimacy.

I also acknowledged my unknown grief had straddled my emotions, my thoughts, and my feelings. It had also vastly limited my mind, my experiences, and expressions in my relationships. I began to understand that I needed to heal my grief and release my emotional voids before experiencing my unique sense of intimacy. I found this realisation to be intensely painful as I feel I was fooled by myself, by my smugness for so long because I ignorantly believed in a conditioned intimacy and a conditioned love.

My sensory awareness of the Light, of my higher self, grew and expanded. It allowed me to sense Light and unconditional love from a new perspective. The truth of Light nurtured my self-acceptance, self-confidence, and self-respect. I began to believe that I could trust myself entirely in what I was trying to achieve in my healing intention. As I accepted my truth as absolute tangible truth, I fully accepted Light and God's unconditional love as an integral part of me. As I grew stronger in my awareness of Light, I began to see that I no longer looked outward to crave other people's intimacy. I began to understand the intimacy I had wanted in the past was a perceived longing of a 'want' that was an insatiable desire within me. It reflected the void created by me in my acceptance of conditional love.

I became conscious of the other grief and unhappy layers that I had never accepted within my mind. I sensed the excruciating pain I felt when my mother died. The pain was overwhelming because it manifested in my healing to be the pain of a broken heart. I recognised the pain I felt at the loss of my home and my family when my father ejected me from it when I was a teenager. The separation from my mother at this young age was a trauma I had denied within me.

I sensed the grief at losing my school friends, the precious bonds from my childhood that I had never acknowledged in my mind.

I sensed the loss of my father when he died. I sensed the loss of my relationships with my siblings, as different emotions separated and alienated us from each other.

Grief was driving my mind unknowingly, invisibly in darkness. It has taken me many years of challenging my thinking to gain these insights and release my grief and recognise my pain.

In this darkness of my bravado mind, I saw I was reckless in my thoughts. I saw my defensive thinking. I was defensive of my husband and children. I challenged any person that I thought didn't respect or value them. I was defensive of myself in every aspect of my interactions. Defence and defending behaviour were honourable and acceptable to me back then, as I perceived such conduct as the strength of my mind.

2. How I used my Senses to Interpret and Build the Thoughts in My Inner Mind.

I saw how my senses interpreted my parents' minds automatically. I saw that I tuned into their whole minds, not just what they wanted me to know. I sensed what they felt. I sensed their thoughts. I sensed what they chose not to say. I saw that I cultivated my intuition into my truth that was the basis of all my emotions. I saw that I ignored my intuitive interpretations and silently, negatively, automatically took them to be my learned truth. For example, I interpreted their silences as a slight against me. I sensed their silent blame, but I accepted it as their blame on me. I sensed their fear of failure or their potential failure, and I instantly made it a fear of failure in my mind.

I now recognise that I silently cultivated this genius, complicated process in my mind to please my parents. I can see I desperately wanted to fit with them, to feel their love and to know they loved me. I truly believed that they knew me as I thought I knew them. I honestly thought I knew what they wanted from me that would please them. Without a doubt, I loved my parents, and I thought they loved me in the same way. Now I can see that my intuited inner mind's development was a silent, unsaid invisible creation. My parents did not know or recognise this hidden unknown me. They were not conscious of how and why I worked so diligently – which was to please them. They could not know how I silently built my mind based on what I had believed they wanted from me. They had no idea of the distress I felt to appear 'normal' to them. They did not know that I needed to feel their love. I needed to hear their approval of me and know their acceptance of me. From my current perspective, I can identify how and why I became angry with them automatically, unconsciously, and subconsciously because they did not recognise my enormous internal efforts to be a good daughter. They never acknowledged how hard I worked for them. I never heard them say that they approved of me. I never heard them say they were happy with me. I never heard them say that they loved me. I can recognise that this silent communication between us was their dynamic of control. I can also see that their silence flipped in my mind to develop into the silent ignition of my automatic unknown, invisible bravado anger that protected me from my truth which revealed my feelings of being unwanted.

3. My Intuited interpretations of the Power of the Family Dynamic of Thinking.

I believed my father was a reliable, dominant provider in my immature perceptions. I imitated and adapted the father's survival-based thinking to build a similar strength in my mind. I perceived my mother as weak and powerless. I interpreted these perceptions in several ways from her behaviour. The behaviour I sensed was mostly her actions and interactions with my father. She was the silent one. She never argued with him in front of the family. Yes, I recognised her face after they had a row. I saw her face when they weren't arguing. I knew her face when she looked out at the faraway mountains.

We communicated freely with her, and it was through her that we related to our father.

I can see I automatically accepted my father's projected thoughts that became my thoughts, my way of thinking. I saw that since he was the strong one, I automatically accepted she was the weak one. I remember thinking this weakness was not part of my personality or mind. I had sensed that my father did not like weakness, and I knew it displeased him. I discarded my 'weakness' automatically to please him.

In my mind, I copied my father's opinions and his behaviour towards my mother. Like him, I had no value on my mother. I didn't distinguish her from her work or her role. I assumed I had a relationship with her. I held an assumed entitlement to her. She was an automatic, permanent extension of my life that was indistinguishable from whom I was then. I had never envisaged my life without her. I had never looked beyond her in my life. I had accepted her presence in my life automatically in my immature, childlike way. I genuinely did not know I loved her as much as I did. It was after I revealed my grief that I found the pain I felt at her loss. I also got a sense of the love she had for all of us, her children. In this love, she stands out as a beacon of unconditional love, which she shares with the whole family. I sense now she is the essence of pure Light.

4. My Intuited Inherited Interpretation of the Family Dynamic of Thinking.

I recognised I had automatically intuited the inherited span of the family dynamic into my mind by not questioning it and by accepting the mindset of my family dynamic as my mind. I recognised past generations' influences as the invisible yet prominent energies of my irrational thoughts or emotions that I needed to identify, detach from, and face their challenges from within my thoughts and feelings.

5. My interpretation of Society's Intuitive Dynamic of Thinking.

The barrier-based perspectives of my bravado mind connected automatically to similar perspectives in the external collective consciousness. These perspectives were the invisible intuitive mirrors of comfort magnets I sought when I engaged with friends, co-workers, and my husband and in all my relationships of love. I saw I responded to what I liked or thought wouldn't hurt me because they seemed 'nice' and sociably acceptable. In my Light awareness, I never use the word 'nice' to describe anyone. When I hear someone else describe a person as 'nice,' I instantly engage my detachment boundaries. 'Nice' is a term that describes a trap filled with different ingredients of mind games, of polished familiar manipulation, lies, betrayal, and judgement and, particularly, control. The smiling presentable face of 'nice' is the honey that lures another person into its mental trap. It is not the 'nice' person who feels the betrayal and abuse when a relationship breaks down. It is the trusting person who engaged and believed in the 'nice' person without exercising their boundaries for protection that suffers.

6. My Interpretation of Society's Inherited Dynamic of Thinking.

As a human being, I felt I was stuck with my mind and my brain, which I could not change. I often asked myself why my brain wasn't brainy like other brains in my family or classes. Now I recognise my automatic acceptance of society's prevailing opinions that the mind is the brain which is the person, and the person is the brain which is the mind.

Our culture reflects their different hierarchies of power by acknowledging and rewarding the brightness of the power of people's minds and their brains.

We assume our identity by listening to and allowing these bright people to tell us we are not as bright as them and are therefore lesser than them. The hierarchy of said dominant society rejects or dismisses us as being stupid. We are recognisable because we languish on the lower steps of society's authorities. Mostly we are invisible or hidden underneath the piles of intellectually bright people scampering for power. They mark us with their shoe prints as they stand on our backs and shoulders to dance their pirouettes of successful and outstanding achievements.

How does this happen? Who developed the thinking and power structures that are so corrosive to the human mind's development?

7. My Interpreted Intuited Religious Thinking.

I saw my internal mind aligned perfectly with the structures of my religious teachings that automatically created my religious dynamic of thinking. In my understanding of them, these religious structures were dark, painful, ritualistic, and rigid in their themes. I intuitively learned to escape the harsh laws of suffering by fleeing mentally into the alternative realities of my daydreams, into the realms of the eternity of my religious thinking, into the lives of my idols. I saw my patterns of thought permitted me to believe that what I lacked in my current life, Jesus would provide for me in heaven when I died. I can see that this thinking was a powerful tool of irresponsibility in my mind that helped me to remain powerless and passive, mentally, emotionally, and physically.

8. My Interpretation of my Religious Intuited Feelings.

The revelation of the invisible intuited, unknown inner me on my knees, head bowed, hands clasped in intense prayer was the image of me that I did not know or recognise. When I saw it in meditation, I recognised it was a significant aspect of the internal victim-me. In this intuited image, I was without any sense of purpose or intention for a better me. In that image, I felt my silent suffering, fear, and anxiety. I saw I had learned not to look up because I didn't want to recognise difficult or painful situations that were challenging for me to understand and that would add to my pain and fear. I knew that if I had acknowledged what I saw, I was too frightened to say what I thought.

However, my mind was confident that I was right in my thinking and my humility. I was right in my acceptance of the pain that I was offering up to God. I was right in my prayers to God. I was right in my prayers to the Mother of God, the saints, and angels.

I saw I had used my interpreted religious teaching against my core self. I saw I needed the pain of my religion, I needed to feel pain, I needed the comfort of pain, and I needed to accept suffering. I needed the painful burden of both my life and Jesus' life to feel normal.

I revealed I had accepted the suffering of Jesus as the love of Jesus. His pain was the love I learned to seek. It became the intuitive automatic way I loved myself, how I loved God, how I loved others. I expected love from people in the same burdened way, otherwise I did not recognise their love.

9. My Intuited Family Dynamic of Automatic Behaviour.

When I began revealing my mind's contents, the most significant insight revealed my intuitive ability to interpret. In the main, I had negatively interpreted the family dynamic of thinking and feeling in fear, and as a result, I developed a negative void of lacking in my mind. For example, I revealed that the lack of value I had on myself was linked back to how I had interpreted my father's opinion of me and the lack of value he had for me. This insight followed on to reveal many other patterns of lacking that related to my relationship with my father. My intuitive interpretations developed in my mind as a lack of self-care, self-tolerance, self-acceptance, self-validation, self-recognition, self-responsibility, and self-respect. I had no awareness or knowledge of this lacking in my mind, which meant I was ignorant of a considerable part of my mind.

I discovered many of my perspectives spun in the different aspects of my learning and knowledge automatically. This spinning permitted me to survive any challenges that came from outside relationships or events.

For example, when I went to the gym to get fit, I approached my gym from my current adult perspective. I instantly felt exhausted just by looking at my programme. I tried to push through this exhaustion, but I always gave up. I also tried yoga, and during many years of practice, I always felt my body's stiffness and its resistance to stretch. I was determined to loosen my muscles and joints, but I gave up because of the pain I felt and the belief that yoga could not help me cope with my pain.

I remember when I began my walking routine, I was determined to succeed. Light intuitively urged me to walk faster during my routine, but always my sense of exhaustion held me back. My walk of purpose to exercise became a stroll. I recognised that I had spent a great deal of my adult life managing my exhaustion.

One day during one of my swim exercises, a memory of an experience of distance flashed into my mind. I saw myself at the age of four or five with my sisters walking to school. About halfway, I wanted to stop and go home, I was tired, but my sisters carried and dragged me the rest of the way to school.

Until I had this insight, which was only very recently, I associated the exhaustion with my weight, my body ageing, and old age generally. When I transmuted this exhausted child learning within my mind, it became more comfortable for me to experience exercise without feeling the invisible learned exhaustion. As I detached and transmuted this learning in my mind, I analysed all the sensations that the young child-me had felt and learned. I can recall my sisters' frustrations with me as they told me impatiently that we had come too far for us to go back home. I heard their persistent urgings for me to keep going as it was only a short distance further. These urgings repeatedly echoed in my mind as I saw the child-me on what seemed to be an endless road struggling to finish the journey to school.

In my child-mind, I learned the exhaustion of distance from the perspective of an upset, small child. I recognised that I regressed to this learning automatically when I, as an adult, challenged myself to exercise. This learned exhaustion weighed heavily but invisibly in my mind and manifested in my body as I struggled with breathing and painful, tired, stiff, and frozen limbs.

From my Light awareness, I have created boundaries. I have learned to live my life without pain. I have learned balance and harmony. I have learned how to self-validate. I have found self-acceptance. I have developed self-control and self-discipline in my mind. I have learned responsibility, self-respect, strength, and courage. I have become gracious in my acceptance of my inspired and intuited thoughts. For this reason, I know that the relationship I have between my Light awareness and my childlike bravado mind is the most critical in existence for me.

Cutting of the Ties Therapy

As my confidence in my awareness grew, I felt prompted by Light to cut ties with my father.

Cutting of the ties is the ultimate, potent, energy-based healing therapy because it permits a person to alter their mind's vibrations and dynamic. It means a person can create an entirely new perspective based on the awareness of Light's boundaries.

To fully participate in the cutting the ties' session, a person must be aware of their connection to their unique Light. Through their perspective of Light, they will reveal their spiritual wounds and controlling emotions. Their Light awareness strengthens and supports the resolve of the person cutting the ties. This resolve requires immense self-discipline to adhere to the rules of the therapy.

A person must accept and understand that there is a universal difference between their Light awareness and their learned bravado mind. It is also essential for the person to understand that a self-created mind cannot be healed or altered from the same mind's perspective.

The process of cutting the ties reveals and releases the invisible, unknown mental barriers contained in the bravado mind. At the same time, it expands and reveals the Light awareness of the heart chakra, the higher self.

The cutting of the ties is a compelling experience for a person, and it facilitates the journey into self-awareness and self-empowerment.

The invisible, unknown ties are the unrecognised mental barriers the average mind perspective works through each second and minute of the day and night. These mental barriers glue people together unknowingly and invisibly in relationships, particularly with family members and long-term relationships. The mental barriers also maintain the hierarchy that upholds families, society and religions.

It is essential to understand the chakras and the chakra system. They are the vital elements that support the mind's structure that contains their uniquely interpreted mental, emotional, and spiritual wounding. The spiritual wounding and the learned suffering are the sources for chronic pain within the mind. It is this wounding and suffering that the cutting of the ties therapy releases.

The mental pain, the perceived fear of pain, the physical pain, and the projected pain, I call sensory pain. Accumulatively, I call them chronic pain. The chest area is the most sensitive part of the body as it contains the heart chakra, the invisible centre of the chest, the physical heart, and the respiratory system. Human behaviour automatically attaches painful feelings and emotions to the physical heart and clogs up the respiratory system with mental barriers of learned blocking fear and painful emotions.

The heart chakra is the invisible sensory point or centre that interprets and accepts all this sensory pain. The heart chakra's sensitivity instantly feels the penetrative opinions or the violating projected emotions, or the silent, angry thoughts, the violent words and deeds projected by others to be immediately and profoundly wounding to a person. This wounding does not kill a person physically or mentally, but it does invisibly crucify a person – in their inner mind and internal organs. The infliction of invisible, paralysing, spiritual wounds registers and remains in the organs that generate pain, fear, and dread internally in a person's inner mind.

A person's bravado mind perspective is also capable of self-violation and self-wounding internally in the inner mind in the same way. The reveal of these chronic spiritual wounds manifests during the cutting of the ties therapy. They are invisible and unknown to a person's perspective, and eventually manifest in the physical body as chronic diseases. The heart's typical chronic disorders are coronary artery disease, heart attack, abnormal heart rhythms or arrhythmias, heart failure, heart valve disease, congenital heart disease, and heart muscle disease.

The respiratory system's typical chronic disorders are asthma, chronic obstructive pulmonary disease, chronic bronchitis, emphysema, lung cancer, and pneumonia.

General subdued feelings of melancholy, sadness, and sorrow also manifest mentally from this chronic sensory and spiritual pain. We recognise these feelings and emotions as anxiety or depression that quietly fuel the irrational thoughts that manifest for no apparent reasons in a person's mind.

Spiritual wounds manifest from each of the chakras showing the appropriate weapons of wounding that belong to that part of the body. But, the heart chakra presents the most defined spiritual injuries and weapons. Typically, they show as a stabbed heart, a festering sore heart, a pierced heart, a broken heart, a blade in the heart, a sword in the heart, a spear through the back into the heart, or a heavy stone lying on the heart.

In my own experience, it was a man's arm that manifested. The elbow was protruding outwards from my chest. The fist was clutching my physical heart and respiratory system in a strong, masculine grip.

The type of weapons used in the wounding indicates which era inflicted the wound. For example, a spear usually means a previous ancient existence automatically inherited from the previous generation. The blade's quality will also indicate how long it has existed in the person's heart. The blade represents a physical, mental, or spiritual wounding that portrays betrayal by a close relative or friend. Betrayal is one of the most potent spiritual crimes anybody can commit against another person.

I wish to explain that the cutting of the ties is a rigorous therapy because it shifts the balance of power and powerlessness within the person's mind electing to cut ties. It can mean changes in the person's mind, their relationship with themselves, and other people, particularly with people within their family dynamic.

For this reason, it must be sought and engaged solely for healing and evolution purposes and not for any irresponsible or combative purposes. The danger of using the cutting of the ties therapy for combative reasons can threaten the sanity or the balance of the mind in the person who is cutting ties.

In my healing career, I have heard many insights into how people abuse the cutting of the ties therapy. I have heard many people give their automatic reasons for the cutting of the ties, particularly revenge. I have listened to people's understanding of their engagement and application to undergo the cutting of ties therapy. I have heard that individuals have cut ties with aspects of their minds. As I sit and listen, I shudder at the ignorance that people have of such an inspiring, empowering, enlightening therapy. I compare their actions of cutting their ties to a heart surgeon operating on his own heart while under anaesthetic.

My Journey into the Cutting of the Ties

I clearly remember the day when Sara suggested to me that I should cut ties with my father. I shivered in every part of my body. I believe a truth dawned within me that inspired me to understand I was a victim of my family dynamic in my sacrificial thinking. I instinctively knew that I could no longer deny this truth.

Sara was a senior spiritual healer. I knew she was a fantastic support to us, the aspiring healers in the centre. She was a recognised expert on the subject of cutting the ties. I booked an appointment with her. I began my first engagement of a therapy that was a first experience for me, and I am sure it was a first for my family. I had a limited understanding of cutting the ties at this point in my development. Nevertheless, I was about to embark on a journey to cut ties between my father and myself. I had no idea of the depth of healing and clarity that this simple therapy was about to unfold into my mind.

Sara explained the process of cutting the ties. She told me the therapy worked in a meditative state, and she asked me to research my relationship with my father. She said it would take two weeks to grasp this relationship and understand the seriousness of my intention to cut the ties.

Occasionally during those two weeks, I felt weird. I often sensed a fleeting feeling of freedom within me. I was conscious of the automatic comfort zone I associated with my father. I was feeling fearful of losing him entirely. He was the only father I had. I knew I was deliberately seeking a release from him and his control.

I didn't know if there were consequences to my actions. I didn't know how my feelings towards my father would pan out afterwards.

I was finally ready to let go of the negative influences in my mind, which I attributed to my father. Sara was comfortable proceeding with the therapy. I began to settle into my meditative state. I was agitated and conscious of feeling more anxious and burdened in my mind than usual. Sara told me that the ties would manifest from each of the chakra points in my aura, which connected me to a relevant chakra point in my father's aura. I began the process of cutting the ties.

For example, the first obstacle that manifested for me was in my heart chakra. I felt all my senses pull towards my heart chakra. I saw a man's arm with its elbow protruding outward, and it was clutching the inside of my chest and my physical heart in a tight fist. I sat in disbelief. I felt stunned at what I was seeing and feeling. I was ashamed because I did not want to say what I was seeing. I wished and prayed it would go away, disappear. I began to sob as I felt the intensity of the pain from this clenched fist.

Sara was very patient with me as it took a long time to release the imprint of this obstacle from my upper body. Unfortunately, I cannot remember all the obstacles I worked through that day, although I remember the other chakras were not as intense.

I was astonished at the hidden, unknown barriers of emotional, mental and spiritual pain and distress I was carrying in my mind. I was shocked at the intensity of pain that rose within me. I sobbed at the realisation of how damaged I was in every conceivable way within me that I had not known existed.

Afterwards, I felt strange. I felt drained. I felt exhausted. I knew I had made a difference within because I felt lighter in myself. I thought I had released something, though I didn't know what exactly.

Sara suggested that I go home, rest for a couple of days and allow my newfound awareness and sense of release and freedom to grow and manifest within me. She also suggested that I not reflect on any of the obstacles that I had released because it was possible to re-engage their energy vibration in my thoughts and re-create them. It took a week or so for me to begin to feel better. Many months later, I allowed myself to re-examine the obstacles that revealed to me that day.

Around this time, I happened to have an unscheduled conversation with my mentor. I casually mentioned to him that I had cut ties with my father. I told him I was a little nervous within myself as I felt I was waiting for something to fall in my mind, drown me or some form of an eruption to occur within me. I can now reflect and recognise that I was automatically fearful of regressing to somewhere in my mind that I didn't want to go. He told me he was confident about the work I was doing on myself. He said he felt I had sufficiently grown within myself not to regress in my thoughts or to re-engage old habits. He reassured me that I was on the right path and that it was ok to continue my healing.

Many more months lapsed. I eventually sat down with my healer friend for hours, and we thrashed out the cutting of the ties therapy. I tried to dig into it to find new and identifiable boundaries that allowed me into a fuller understanding and a deeper meaning to the personal obstacles that manifest for people during the therapy sessions.

I think the symbol that had me riding the crest of the wave of curiosity was my symbol of the man's elbow protruding from my heart chakra. Since the cutting of the ties with my father, it was always in my mind. I could not dismiss it. I could not push it aside and pretend that I hadn't seen it. I could not pretend that it had not manifested as a massive crucifying barrier for me in the most sacred place within me, my heart chakra.

The explanations I received from other healers were not enough to satisfy me. I drew the image, and I looked at it. I studied it. And I looked at it again. I stared at it, and very slowly, an understanding grew within my awareness that satisfied me. I started to grasp that I had not just cut physical ties with my father. I had cut ties with his dynamic of thought that included his inherited wounded mindsets from his ancestors that stretched back through the centuries. I had indeed cut ties with my father and his mind, but more importantly, I had cut ties with the father aspect I had created in my mind.

For the first time in my life, I acknowledged and accepted my father's influence on my mind. I had not been aware of the powerful connection between our minds at that stage in my development. I was not aware of how this connectivity worked. I found it as I became aware of my inability to make choices or decisions in my mind. I grew aware of my automatic anger. I became aware I was not living life. I became aware I was only living my life by imitating his way of living. The reveal of the father aspect of my mind showed me that I automatically and conditionally loved. I lived through my perception of how I understood my father had loved and lived, how society in general loved and lived, and the entitled way they wanted me to love them back in return.

I began to understand that the symbol of the man's elbow protruding from my heart chakra was a symbol of how I had shaped my mind, so that I could survive. The protruding man's elbow was my interpretation of my father's strength, his power in the shape of my father's arm. The clenched fist was my interpretation of the father's control, power, and dominance in how he shaped my thoughts and thinking to the detriment of my feelings and mind.

I created the sensory and spiritual pain, and my father's relationship supported me in that pain. It was the male vice-like grip of control and force of power I engaged within my mind. This grip kept me mostly ignorant of my feelings of goodness, intimacy, joy, and my core feelings of unconditional love.

I cried for a long time as I began to understand who I was inside of me, in my mind, and how lost and broken I was.

As I accepted this truth, I recognised that I created my mind in imitation of male thinking. I asked Light how my mind had been created in such an alien way of thinking and learning. After all, I am not male. I am female. How had I become that symbol of maleness in my mind?

I was shocked to understand that it was from and through this negative invisible, unknown male barrier within my mind that I loved my husband and my children. I was horrified to accept I was connecting to my outside world through the same symbol of male thinking. This interpreted symbol of masculine strength was understood and perceived from a perspective that continued into adulthood. I can identify the continuing revelation of other mental male-based barriers and their subsequent releases within my mind from cutting ties with my father. I can also identify how these releases had a direct effect on the vibrations of my mind. From this action – the cutting of the ties – I began to understand the reflective mindset. I accepted insights into how I built my mind.

I began to recognise my father's physical pain had become my pain in my physical body.

My back ached and stiffened. My joints in my fingers and toes had started to freeze. I started to understand the control and power the collective consciousness had on my thinking. To me, this thinking felt it was the strength of my mind.

I also began to see that as I grew from a child, my older sisters and my older brother were very authoritative and influential in my life. They were not just my sisters and brother, but they seemed to be a combination of parental control over me. I cannot recall either of my parents correcting their authority or their parenting over me. It meant that not only had I absorbed into my mind the imprint of my parents' authority and control, but I had also absorbed my siblings' imprints of their interpretations of their parenting that became my mind also. I grew in my mind to become a combination of my interpretation of my parents' minds and my older siblings' minds. I passed this learning on to my younger siblings as my authority, my parenting, my control. I cannot remember if my parents ever corrected me in my parenting of my younger siblings.

As my relationship with my father revealed and the detachment process deepened, images began to manifest

in my awareness and my dreams that revealed the damaged child aspects of my mind. I saw the hurt child, the
pleasing child, the sick child, the exhausted child, the
lonely child, the fearful child, the worried child, the angry
child, the anxious child, the alone child. There were repeated images of a young girl working as an adult works.

My higher self, or my Light awareness, intuited me
to learn to listen to my inner voice. By listening to and
hearing my unique intuitive voice, I began to distinguish
the father voice in my thoughts.

As I identified his voice, I began to feel his anger
churn in my stomach. I began to feel and hear the echo
of his criticism as my self-criticism in my thinking. My
critical voice was harsh, as harsh as my father's voice. It
had an even more damaging impact on my vulnerabilities
than my father's criticism.

I began to identify his dismissive voice in my thoughts,
which I adapted as my voice in my automatic dismissive
thoughts and behaviour.

I began to remember incidents from my childhood
when his expectations and demands ensured the loss of
my childhood innocence in playfulness and freedom. I
am sure this is true for all my siblings. As growing children, we all worked hard on the farm, especially during
the summer and autumn. We cut and stacked the turf,
sowed and picked potatoes, saved the hay, packed the hay
barns, picked vegetables, picked stones and weeds from
the meadows. This work was in addition to the regular
chores we did on the farm. I started to see how, as a child,

I imitated him. I sensed his power, and I imitated it. I mirrored his actions. I mimicked his strengths. I echoed his opinions automatically. I imitated his behaviour. I recognised how I gloried in my perceptions of his unrelenting expectations of me.

I can now see that it did not matter what task or job he asked me to do. I made sure I did it right and even better than it was done previously. I tried to ensure my younger siblings did their jobs right.

The combination of working hard and my physical growth helped me to feel strong mentally, which fuelled the bravado attitude in my mind as I grew into a teenager. I can see stages in my thinking where I recognised his weakness and I stored it away in my mind. I was very conscious of not liking my father's actions and his behaviour. I felt I wanted more from him, not just for me, but for my mother and my siblings.

I recognised when my parents placed heavy adult responsibilities firmly on my incredibly young older siblings' shoulders. As they grew and my parents added more children to the family, they passed on their interpretations and thinking of these responsibilities, which in turn, I passed on to my younger siblings.

I started to understand that this was automatic learning with little or no application of self-awareness required by me. It ejected my childhood innocence and child awareness into an adult perspective. As I advanced into adulthood, it left the growing child-me, unknowingly physically and mentally overburdened by my child's mind acceptance of this overburden. I began to see the lack of individual responsibility in my thoughts. I also saw my interpreted perceptions of the collective irresponsibility's in my parents' minds, in their relationships with their children, and the ongoing relationships between the growing children. I accepted that the lack of individual responsibility was a severe culprit in the corrosion of my self-esteem and self-confidence, which I now see I lacked as a child and as an adult.

I saw my ability to self-loathe. I recognised my shame that was driving my resistant, defensive thinking and behaviour. I understood my unworthiness within me as I found my father's voice telling me to do things for other people and not ask them for money.

For a while, it seemed I was in the reveal of the spin of my buried pain that was caught up and contained in that tight fist of male power that held my heart. It became my quest to unclench the fist and remove its grip from my heart and respiratory system.

I began to understand that my father's relationship with each of my siblings and me was fraught with frustrations, fear, anger, and other anxieties. I can also see that my siblings have individually cultivated their father aspects within their mind dynamics. I can see that our unique ability to interpret his mind was the fundamental difference between us in our thoughts and our feelings.

His mental legacy to his sons and daughters, which was our automatic mental birthright, became an inheritance of a powerful yet angry, narrow, self-sufficient, survival-driven mind based on emotions of unconscious fear and anger. Because it is automatically our legacy and our inheritance, I didn't question my mind. My mind felt normal to me because it was me.

I found the reveal of my siblings' parenting challenging to recognise, accept, comprehend, heal, and transmute. For example, my eldest sister automatically carried the tremendous burden and responsibility of parenting that I could recognise when I began to unravel our relationship. She was a combination of both my parents in my bravado thinking and dependencies. It was her I looked to when I needed coping skills. I copied her when I was struggling to cope with my relationship. I copied her when I fought to become a good mother. I trusted my children would be safe with her. I saw I relied on her for a sense of strength in the same way I had mirrored my parents in my need to survive.

Now I understand that I loved her in a childlike, dependent way that became an even greater need in me with my mother's premature death. How unfair was I, the big bravado person, silently burdening her in this way? How unfair was I to add to her responsibilities of her own immediate family? How unfair was I not to appreciate the added responsibilities she took on without question when she cared unconditionally for my father and aunt? How blind was I not to see the exertions she was making mentally to cope with all her responsibilities? Who was I that I could not support her? Who was I, this dependent child-like adult, looking to her to parent and help me? All the while, I was masquerading as a successful, responsible parent in my own life.

I also held one of my sisters on a pedestal of mental power. I relied on her approval of me from a young age. She approved of my looks. She approved of my humour. I assumed she approved of me. I relied on her for my answers. I accepted her answers as truth, as fact. Her voice became a parenting voice somewhere in my mind. I slavishly loved her. For a long time, I was blind and deaf to any of her vulnerabilities and weaknesses. I could only see the power and the good of the woman. When I perceived her pain, I took it as my own and as my fault, my weakness when our relationship clashed.

It took me many years of spiritual healing to accept that these people were sisters to me and had no other responsibility towards my family or me.

I have an older brother absent in my life for as long as I can remember due to asthma that choked and paralysed him while he lived on the farm. He was not absent physically. However, during the summer and autumn months, he could not contribute to the farm work because of his allergies. We did not know he suffered from allergies then. I just knew that he was sick again. The others in the family picked up the slack and had to work harder.

There was another significant yet unknown presence in my life that was absent. That presence was of an older baby boy sibling between my brother and me that had died in a miscarriage. That miscarriage had a significant effect on my mother's health as she very nearly died. She was ill in bed for months afterwards. My older siblings must have perceived and understood the threat of their mother dying as massive fears in their minds. I believe that this invisible traumatic fear of near-death became embedded in my mother's mind and our family dynamic automatically from that time. My older sisters, who were at particularly tender ages, had to become parents to each other and to my older brother, who was only a toddler at that time.

My parents must have hidden their fears about her illness, and they felt there was no need for them to explain or comfort or reassure their children. I understand how that triggered great fears in their children's minds. This lack of communication held negative triggers for all the children, but it mainly affected my brother's mind. I believe it manifested for him physically in his asthma attacks. I remember he often collapsed into unconscious states many times, especially when he struggled for breath. I remember my father kneeling beside him for what seemed like hours, calling his name repeatedly, asking him to stay with him and not to die. During these difficult times, one of my older sisters was sent out to our neighbours to phone a doctor. My other sister gathered up the younger ones, and we would disappear up the land and find ways to pass the time until we thought it was safe to return.

As a growing girl, I dreamed and longed for times when he would be better. My mother often told me that he would grow out of his asthma. I had deadlines in my head that I longed to reach so he could be a normal brother and no longer have asthma, and we all could begin to feel normal. It never happened. My brother's health only improved when he left the farm and began to work in the city.

I discovered my mother's dreamlike avoidance in my mind. Her passive opinion of my brother's illness became a coping mechanism that I imitated in my mind. I avoided decisions, drama and conflict. That was my way of coping with challenges to my 'peaceful life.' As I matured in my life and as dramatic events happened in my adult relationships that were glaring red flags, signals of danger, I ignored them. Instead of taking action, I dreamed passively of the future when things would be better, and I would feel better.

My relationships also mirrored my father's relationship with his son. I saw my father's patience when my brother was unconscious, and he wouldn't allow my brother to die. At the same time, when my brother's health was ok, my father and my brother did not get on. In my relationships, I accepted disrespectful behaviour as normal behaviour to me. I didn't ask for improved behaviour. I took the disrespect, hoping or assuming it would improve.

I prayed that people would see their wrong thinking, their controlling ways with me. I wanted them to see their manipulating ways. I wanted them to treat me properly.

It seemed that my prayers for a better life went unanswered by God. I waited and watched the same decisions continuously repeated in my life that eventually alienated me in my relationships. I had to face these challenges myself. I had to ask for better treatment and behaviour in my relationships.

It was the cutting of the ties that revealed these aspects of my mind that helped me to heal and close the emotional and spiritual wounds in my mind. Eventually, I began to feel healthy, feel my courage, feel my self-respect, feel my confidence, and feel my self-esteem.

I know that if I didn't explore spiritual healing and the cutting of the ties with my father, I would have lived in ignorance of these insights and empowered healings. I eventually found the courage to accept that I needed to face and recognise my mother aspects within my thoughts and feelings. I realised that I had been avoiding dealing with my mother influences.

My healing revealed the precious protective layers of defensiveness I had put in place in my bravado mind to protect my relationship with my mother. I, the daughter, the mother, the wife, the sister, always protected my relationship with her in my thoughts. I desperately needed to preserve my memories of her to continue my automatic invisible relationship with her. This relationship with my mother existed for most of my adult life until I began to change it. Eventually, I recognised the automatic blame I carried towards my father for all my mother's ailments and even for her early death.

I can recall how I felt when my mentor told me I should cut ties with her. I found it particularly challenging as my resistance and defensiveness kicked in. I recognised the suggestion had triggered an enormous fear – a fear of loss and a fear of pain – that was weighing heavily on my physical heart. I recognised the fear in my anxiety that I would lose my feelings for her which I had harboured and held close since she had passed on. I saw she was a hugely important part of me, subconsciously, unconsciously, and consciously. She was a massive presence in my life without my knowing it or without my ever becoming conscious of her value as a mother.

After that initial ban of me from our home as a teenager by my father, she had kept up communication with me. We often wrote to each other, and eventually, I relented to come home and accept a reconciliation of sorts with my father without anyone saying anything. I facilitated that reconciliation with my father mainly to please my mother. On reflection, I can see that I used every opportunity to come home to her after that visit. I would help her by doing jobs around the house to be with her, near her.

However, I am ashamed to say I thought she was weak in another aspect of my mind. Her health was not good. She was always working. I could never understand why she could not challenge my father to improve her life. It seemed to me she never challenged my father's decisions. She just accepted them and never asserted her wishes or her desires, even though we often discussed her dreams. I discovered that her way had also become my way of surviving in my life and in my marriage.

I figured out other similarities in our relationships. The main similarity between our minds was both of our desires to live a quiet life. This insight was significant to me. It left me in a state of shock as I had spent most of my life trying not to have my mother's lifestyle. I had worked extremely hard not to be a weak person. This insight alone was a very definite reason for me to begin cutting ties with her. I did not want to influence either my daughter or my son's behaviour in that passive way – unconsciously, subconsciously, or consciously. My most sincere wish for them is that they become aware, strong individuals living their lives to their unique purpose and intention.

To heal my relationship with my mother completely, I had to find the mother aspect of my mind I had interpreted and developed into my bravado mind. I had to find her in my thoughts, emotions, feelings, and religious beliefs.

I started by finding my perceived and actual weaknesses in my thinking. I had to find and engage with my emotions, no matter how dense or painful. I had to find behaviour I had rejected or deliberately shed from my mind in my efforts not to be weak or be like my mother. I had to find my heart and all its heartache. I had to heal and release the suppressed, intense pain I felt after she died. To do and complete this healing within me, I had to find compassion for myself. I prayed for the courage I needed to survive this healing and not to succumb to my pain.

I relied on Light to help me, even though sometimes I felt it was a fleeting sense of Light. Nevertheless, my acceptance of the Light within facilitated my self-healing. I revealed how I had automatically created different, powerful emotions influenced by my unknown, invisible grief for her. I revealed the mythical relationship I had developed with her in my mind since her death. I saw how guilty I felt because I had rejected her in my automatic childlike way when I decided not to live her life at a young age.

Now I can recognise that I betrayed her. I was ashamed of her. I felt guilty about her life and how hard she had to work. I had to engage these and other emotions through Light to release their relevant pained wounds from my heart.

I recognised, healed, and released betrayal. I found more guilt. I felt hugely responsible for the awfulness of my relationships with my siblings. I felt guilty because I was not present in their lives, which may have helped them have better lives during my prolonged absences.

I felt guilty that I missed milestones in the lives of my siblings' children. I understood that this was my automatic bravado perspective that did not see or accept that these people have their lives, opinions, and truths about our relationships.

When I released my guilt, I found my fear. I had learned that fear in my childhood. I had interpreted that fear as a child. That child did not understand life or how life works from an adult perspective, did not understand feelings and emotions, and that child did not understand the importance of boundaries and personal responsibility. As an adult, I can reflect on my overburdened, accumulative sense of responsibility and duty for others. In my childlike intensity, I believed that I could save, protect, and influence people.

I remain in the healing process with my siblings. Clarity from Light in my thoughts is helping me to understand my responsibilities. Clarity also gives me the courage to reject the projected blame I sense from other people.

I eventually found the courage to cut ties with my mother. I instantaneously sensed freedom and lightness. At the same time, I felt my connection with my mother was different. I realised I had not lost my feelings for her as I had feared, and I now have new sensations that I feel are present in my heart chakra. My awareness of her blends with the Light of my higher self and her presence only manifests at different times during the highly intensive situations in my life. I often sense her presence in my children's lives and the lives of my siblings and their children. These sensations of her presence are of her standing invisibly to honour her family while she emits feelings of joy, pride, excitement and achievement. I can also sense her at times of danger or potential danger.

When I send out Light during absent healing work, she supports me, and we work together. I often sense her encircling arm of support for each of us. She exists in high sensations of Light, though I am unaware of her presence for the most part.

There are occasions when she emerges into my awareness with a blanket of protection. I trust my intuition that the sense of her shield is adequate awareness for me now. I do not need to feel this blanket around me or have no need to own this shield. In other words, I have inspired myself into believing and understanding that this blanket does not need to be any of the comfort pacifiers I used as a child. I am an adult. I am no longer a child with childish wants and needs. I must not regress into childlike thinking to find an identity, a feeling of comfort, security, familiarity, a sense of belonging, and a sense of love.

As I healed and released my passivity, I discovered my automatic habit of accepting the easy way out of life's challenges. For a long time, I could not recognise the inaction of my passivity. I had mixed up this emotional and mental paralysis with an assumed affection, care, love, loyalty, duty, support, and compliance.

I looked under the religious mental shroud of my conformist thinking and the inherited folklore, which I had accepted automatically because my mother told me to. She told us the stories that influenced me in believing and genuinely feeling the rightness and the righteousness that were her truth, which I made to be my truth. I found that my acceptance of religion was similar to her acceptance of religion. I recognised her behaviour in her faith as my behaviour in my faith. As I released my passivity, I saw my need to experience the quiet life as the main reason for practising my religion. I finally found my automatic thinking of 'I have to' or 'we have to' as the mantra that ruled my mind.

In my first reading with my mentor, he channelled the energies of my mother. His interpretation of her message was intensely beautiful for me to hear. She said, "I had to leave this world early. I can do more for you all in my invisible state than I could ever have tried to do if I was alive and physically with you." I believe this to be true. Whenever I get the opportunity, I remind my siblings and their children of this message.

As a daughter, I understand that I loved my mother without question. In our relationship, I felt magnetised to her. I only understood this pull towards her back then in my constant visits home to see her and be with her. Latterly, I see she was a woman of dignity and love. She shared what she had unconditionally. I endeavour to reach her heights of dignity and courage within me as an adult as I began to realise who I am and where I stand in my life.

The healing of this giant aspect of me has been painful and frustrating. With each release, I grow stronger in my heart as our Lights merge and continue to blend into the higher vibrations of Light. I have found my connection, my anchorage to the Light of the universe through her. My Light link is my true inheritance. It is my unique birthright and is my mother's gift to me. I see it was through her Light connection in her heart chakra that my aura was created. From this high point in Light, I travelled into the denseness in my mind to become me, the human being that I am.

I finally detached my consciousness, my mind, from the power of the collective. I focused my intention and my purpose to connect to this anchorage of Light. I have put a structure of boundaries around this Light connection that has allowed me to change, alter, and invent a new mind for myself. My conscious intention to evolve is always building my Light awareness. At the same time, I am consciously healing and releasing my bottomless pit existence of pain. In my Light awareness, I now reach upward to higher vibrations of Light to find my answers. I find I no longer need to regress to the womb, my mother, her heart, or my family dynamic of love and acceptance for me to flourish and to blossom.

During my life, I subconsciously, unconsciously, and consciously tried to fill other people's shoes. I didn't just step into their shoes – I fully accepted the imprint of their minds and their lives as my mental imprint.

As a healing and evolving person, I now accept that I must step into the universe to determine who I am as an individual. I tentatively begin to take these steps as I declare to the world that my insights and my Light awareness are objective, rational, inspirational, and supportive. I share my journey and its oscillations as best I can. As I attempt to take my steps into the universe and Light, each step must be a conscious step taken from a Light perspective.

About the Author

During the late nineties, I was regularly meditating and facilitating meditation groups, so becoming a spiritual healer was a natural progressive step for me to take.

However, I was naïve and ignorant of myself and my mindset, and it took some time before I realised that I could not help other people until I healed myself first. During a dream in 2004, a Spirit handed me a book called the Annals of Healing which he said was for me. I experienced a range of emotions from awe to intrigue to fear. I now realise that Spirit needed to work with my closed mind, but as this book downloaded into my sensory awareness, it became the inspiration and the Light that directed me and helped me heal the darkness in my mind and continues to do so.

It has taken me over twenty years to accept, interpret, and articulate the contents of this book. First, I began writing down the insights into notes that were helping me address the many layers of mental inadequacy and inferiority. I needed to accept and take responsibility for my automatic, religious-based, power-driven mindset. I was coming to my healing career from a mental perspective of survival and felt that I knew all that I needed to know, but

I was ignorant in my mindset. It was my ignorance that clouded and masked my weakness and my pain.

In 2018, I published my first book, My Invisible World, which describes the invisible world of my emotions and Spirit, which were the invisible blocks inhibiting me from my healing intentions. This publication, How I Healed My Mind, describes the revelations I discovered as I went into the darkest part of my mind and uncovered the thoughts controlling me from other people's mindsets and egos. My third book is Healing Through Light Awareness, gives the reader meditations and insights to build a higher awareness of yourself, which I call 'The Light Within'.

I shared the learnings of my healing journey because I feel it is essential to share help and support others on their healing journey. I spent many years struggling in darkness, not knowing I was in mental darkness until I connected to my higher self, my Light within. I hope my books will help anyone searching for truth, insight, awareness of themselves and healing.

Work with Lucy

L ucy Devine is a multi-faceted healer who offers readings to help you with the direction and path of your life and release you from pain and suffering. She also channels healing that will empower you to feel differently about yourself. A severing of the sensory ties therapy can also be included to release you from the mental ties that bind you in painful relationships.

In addition, Lucy offers a meditation designed to shift how you see your world. The healing tools and techniques will change your life by helping you attune with your higher self, also known as "The Light Within." In our busy lives, we often don't pay attention to where we are going, but Lucy assures you that this meditation will help you find yourself on the path of happiness and peace, overcome any obstacle while shifting from pain to love.

With Lucy's support and guidance, you can learn how to establish boundaries with life while letting go of negative emotions and anger. You will feel clearer, lighter, more empowered as you strengthen your inner Light and self-healing awareness.

Lucy can be contacted via email on lucydevine@ gmail.com.

Please Review

Dear Reader,

If you enjoyed this book, would you kindly post a short review on Goodreads or whatever store you purchased to book from? Your feedback will make all the difference to getting the word out about this book.

Thank you in advance.

Printed in Great Britain
by Amazon